TAMING THE
BELOVED BEAST

DANIEL CALLAHAN

TAMING THE
BELOVED BEAST

HOW MEDICAL TECHNOLOGY COSTS ARE DESTROYING

OUR HEALTH CARE SYSTEM

PRINCETON UNIVERSITY PRESS
PRINCETON AND OXFORD

Copyright ©2009 by Princeton University Press
Published by Princeton University Press, 41 William Street,
Princeton, New Jersey 08540
In the United Kingdom: Princeton University Press, 6 Oxford Street,
Woodstock, Oxfordshire OX20 1TR

Cover photo courtesy of Shutterstock

First paperback printing, 2018
Paper ISBN 978-0-691-17799-1

The Library of Congress has cataloged the cloth edition of this book as follows:

Callahan, Daniel, 1930–
Taming the beloved beast : how medical technology costs
are destroying our health care system / Daniel Callahan.
p. ; cm.
Includes bibliographical references and index.
ISBN 978-0-691-14236-4 (hardcover : alk. paper)
1. Medical care, Cost of—United States. 2. Medical technology—
Economic aspects—United States. I. Title.
[DNLM: 1. Biomedical Technology—economics—United States.
2. Health Care Costs—United States. 3. Insurance—
economics—United States. W 74 AA1 V156t 2009]
RA410.53.C353 2009
338.4'33621—dc22   2009001503

British Library Cataloging-in-Publication Data is available

This book has been composed in Aldus

Printed on acid-free paper. ∞

press.princeton.edu

Printed in the United States of America

FOR OUR MANY YEARS TOGETHER

Vincent F. and Yvonne DeBruyn Callahan

William and Patricia Nagle

Michael and Mary Zeik

CONTENTS

This book was completed in the midst of one of the great fiscal crises of American economic history. It is still too early to know what the long-term implications and fallout will be and what it may mean for American health care in particular. How much and what kind of health care reform under a new president and Congress will be possible is now up in the air. The general economic woes surely pushed health care off the front page for a time, and even the presidential candidates had to put it aside for a spell.

Public opinion polls showed a remarkable fluctuation in 2007–2008. For a time they showed that the public saw health care reform, and cost control especially, as a top priority, even more than ending the Iraq war. But by late 2008 it had declined in importance, overshadowed by the larger economic travail. Meanwhile a steady stream of new studies showed the health care system deteriorating: the number of uninsured and underinsured steadily grew, costs continued to rise, employers slowly but steadily cut health care benefits altogether or cut their scope and coverage, out-of-pocket medical expenses continued to rise, and even the reasonably well insured reported financial distress from medical bills.

It was in one sense exhilarating to be writing a book on health care reform at a time when it had become a major domestic issue, even if that status fluctuated from time to time. But it was also distressing. We have a messy system, one ill-designed for reform because of the accretion of assorted interest groups with different agendas and vested interests, an ideologically divided public, and a steady stream of new and expensive technologies added to those already in place. If it is not too difficult to envision an ideal system, and there are many to choose from, it is more difficult to imagine politically just what it will take to put such a system in place. It is hardly less difficult to think of a fully defensible way of dealing with the main ethical dilemma that underlies the management of technology and health care costs: how to persuade the public and health care professionals that any plausible solution will require pain and sacrifice.

But one nice feature of writing on a complex problem was the most satisfying help I received from my colleagues and the research staff of The Hastings Center. They include Alison Jost, who helped me to keep it all straight in too many ways to describe, Gregory Kaebnick and Susan Gilbert, who read the entire manuscript with a sharp editorial eye and charged to assist me in making a sometimes wonkish topic readable and interesting. Jacob Moses and Polo Black chased down a seemingly endless list of obscure references. Mary Crowley provided both substantive and editorial assistance. I was also helped by Blair Sadler, a member of the Center's board of directors and a health policy veteran. My friend Muriel Gillick, the Harvard geriatrician, gave me some prudent advice about setting forth my own views. She's a physician, and I tried, if not always successfully, to be a compliant patient. A special word of thanks must also go to Alain Enthoven, with whom I exchanged many letters on competition in health care. I am afraid I was not persuaded by his arguments, but he was the very model of someone with a superior professional history and uncommon policy experience graciously helping someone with lesser attributes. Finally, I am indebted to my wife Sidney, who had to listen to me talk at inordinate length about a subject that is far afield from her own interests. She was patient and tolerant and had many useful insights.

TAMING THE
BELOVED BEAST

TAMING THE BELOVED BEAST

How Medical Technology Costs are Destroying Our Health Care System

Once again the United States is in the midst of a periodic health care "crisis," one that has emerged about every 15 years since World War II. Once again talk of reform is in the air. Once again public opinion polls show, as they have done for decades, that a strong majority of Americans want universal health care—and also how divided they are about how to get there. Once again the complexity of reform, competing interest groups, and the long-standing resistance to an expanded role for government stand in the way.

Is it different this time? Will reform elude us? Will hopes be dashed? I will not try to prophesy how and when the current struggle will end. I want, instead, to examine a critical variable in any discussion of health care reform, one that is known and visible to health care experts and increasingly by the public but, curiously, politically minimized and evaded as well: the growing cost of medical technology.

In a rare instance of consensus, health care economists attribute about 50% of the annual increase of health care costs to new technologies or to the intensified use of old ones.[1] That annual increase has fluctuated between 7% and 12% a year for many years now, and there is every expectation that it will persist at around 6–7% for the indefinite future. Medicare's cost increases are projected to be 7.4% a year between 2006 and 2017. The health portion of the GDP was 16.3% in 2007 and, at the present rate of increase, will consume 19.5% by 2017.[2] The so-called "magic" of compound interest, much cited as an argument for saving money has, as its nasty twin, rapidly compounded costs. The projections are that the Medicare program will go bankrupt in 10 years or so, and the overall cost of health care will rise from $2.2 trillion in 2007 to over $4 trillion in the next decade or so, an astonishing jump.

That trend is a major contributor to the steady growth of the uninsured, now at 46 million and increasing at the rate of 1 million a year (although 2007 saw a small drop). Costs are no less a contributor to the gradual decline of employer-provided health care (now down to 60%), a reduction in benefits, and an increase in cost-sharing. American health care is increasingly unaffordable for business, for government programs, and for individuals. Despite a popular Medicare program, its beneficiaries, those over 65, will spend an average of $5000 a year of their own money on health care, and some as much as $10,000. Half of all personal bankruptcies in the United States are occasioned by health care debts.

If close to 50% of the cost problem can be traced to medical technology, then one might expect that its costs would occupy a central place in the national debate, and, more specifically, that the various reform proposals now in circulation would give special consideration to the control of technology. The only bright spots have been the inclusion of a $1.1 billion budget item in President Obama's stimulus package for technology assessment (TA), and a smaller amount for information technology (IT). It was immediately attacked by conservatives as a government threat to the doctor-patient relationship. Michael O. Leavitt, the Secretary of the Department of Health and Human Services in the George W. Bush administration, was one of the few people in government to complain vigorously about that neglect. The present growth of health care spending, he said in a September 2008 speech, "could potentially drag our country into a financial crisis that would make our major subprime mortgage crisis look like a warm summer rain."[3] The extensive academic and policy literature that I heavily draw upon in this book tend to treat the cost problem as serious but in far more muted language than that of Secretary Leavitt. His words strike the right note and tone.

One aim of this book is to assess this reticence, but, in brief, the most likely reason is the superelevated stature given to steady medical progress and technological innovation in American culture, medicine, and industry. Progress and innovation seem self-evidently valuable, not to be questioned. The frightening thought that the innovation that has saved so many lives and reduced so much suffering could itself be playing a leading role in our health care discomfort is hard to accept, difficult to talk about openly, and politically controversial. It connotes rationing of medical treatment, limits, and a direct threat to the cherished value of relentless progress against illness and death.

We can readily agree that medical progress and technological innovation have been an enormous human benefit and that many of the readers of this book and I, not to mention millions of others, might not even be alive but for them. They have helped to lower death rates from lethal diseases, extended average life expectancies, relieved us of many forms of physical and mental suffering, and have given us a confidence about living into old age, and a good old age at that, in ways impossible for past generations even to have imagined. Yet if the cost of all those benefits begins to exceed what we can now afford, how do we decide when enough is enough, and just what might count as "enough"? What might be of immense value to us as individuals may not be compatible with an equitable health care system, aiming for a common good, not just the private good.

Is there any wonder, then, that politicians and reformers shy away from the subject? They have trouble enough devising viable system-wide reform proposals without throwing cold water on their own case by dealing directly with costs and technology. They hardly confront the subject at all or, if so, in some soft, nonthreatening way. The most popular line is to pledge a vague reduction of waste and inefficiency, a 30-year-old refrain that is lofty in its rhetoric and devoid of much success. But such a proposal does not get anyone's back up.

Even though technology is the main driver of cost increases, perhaps the reticence to recognize this that I note reflects a belief that technology expenses are important symptoms of the cost problem but not one of its primary underlying pathologies. Often cited are high administrative costs, fee-for-service medicine, a profit-driven private sector, the economic incentives for physicians to use (and misuse) technology, and a medical–industrial complex that finds technology an unparalleled cash cow. Those causes are indeed important, and I discuss them in detail as the book progresses. But I give technology a place of primacy for two reasons. First, I see it as both a cause and an effect, not one or the other. It is a cause because, for most Americans and most doctors, it is the most visible and attractive feature of contemporary medicine and health care. Drugs, surgery, and medical devices of one kind or another are what save our lives and relieve our suffering. And they have a more important role, real and symbolic, in American health care than in most other health care systems. Technology pulls us along, raising our health aspirations as well as our costs. Ezekiel J. Emanuel and Victor R. Fuchs, in a valuable survey article, speak of overutilization of health care procedures, but much of that I call the use, and over-use, of technology. Those are the expensive items but they well bring out how there are other instances of overutilization as well.[4]

Second, technology costs reflect the way our health care system is financed and organized as well as the way our physicians are trained to practice medicine. Even if the many incentives for both the excessive use and misuse of technology as well as its use in cases providing only minimal benefit were all eliminated, the *cost* of technology would still remain a problem because of its very success. Ironically, those very technologies that do work to improve our health and quality of life are increasingly becoming the expensive long-term problem, and that will be the ultimate dilemma for any future health care system.

This book is based on a number of convictions. If costs are not controlled, the health care system will not collapse; it will fall into a gradual decline, with increased inequities, ever more uninsured, and a deterioration of quality. The emergence of a three-tiered system can already be observed. At one level are those with adequate and ample health care coverage, either through private employer-provided coverage or through Medicare, and who are comfortably able to afford co-payments and deductibles. At another level are those who have coverage but are either underinsured or for whom the co-payments and deductibles are economically stressful. Those who must buy their own insurance, or whose employer-provided care does not cover family members, or who face unbearably high costs because of gaps in coverage (many Medicare recipients), fall into this group. It is the second group (estimated at about 25 million) that is fast growing and increasingly touching middle-income people who were previously covered at the first level.[5] At still another tier are those who do not have, or cannot afford, private insurance but must depend on Medicaid, with coverage that is often inadequate. An important way to control costs is to control the use of technology, and the key to doing this is to control physician fees, reimbursements, and acceptable procedures, and to limit industry's excessive influence on the use and marketing of medical technologies.

I can sum up what I want to say in some simple propositions. First, ways must be found to return to more basic levels of medical care for ever more patients (e.g., to emphasize prevention and primary care) and to make it more difficult to receive medical care at the higher levels (e.g., advanced expensive cancer treatments or heart repairs). Second, the priorities for technologically oriented health care should begin with children, remain high with adults during their midlife, and then decline with the elderly. Third, if the medical care received during those first two stages of life is good, the elderly will have a high probability of a good old age even if advanced technologies are less available to them. Fourth, health care cannot be reformed, or costs controlled, without changing some deeply held underlying values, particularly those of unlimited medical progress and technological innovation.

The title of my book, *Taming the Beloved Beast*, is meant to catch the basic dilemma I will be exploring. How do we cope with the much beloved technology of medicine, that brings us uncounted benefits, when that same technology—like a beloved dog who chews up the furniture, scares strangers and small children with his excessively friendly behavior, and is not house broken—begins to create new problems as fast as it can solve old ones. We cannot kill off technological innovation any more than we can comfortably send our dear pet to the vet to be put to sleep. But neither do we have any electrifying ideas about controlling the costs of technology, particularly when, as with our sweet but unruly pet, all of the experts on training dogs (and managing technology) have torn out their hair trying to induce better behavior.

Even if through some miracle we do achieve a universal health care system, we will have an almost impossible time holding on to it without controlling costs in a rigorous way. Steadily growing technology costs, compounded by the retirement of the baby boomers and increased demand on the system, would make it unsustainable. That latter possibility can be seen in European health care systems, struggling to hold on to their universal care in the face of the same kind of cost pressures we face (although doing much better at this than we currently are).

The worst reality of all now is that there are no reliable or seriously envisioned practical and politically acceptable means of managing costs anywhere near the extent necessary. There are, to be sure, many good ideas for controlling escalating costs, but most are theoretical and only speculative. They do not pass the test of "practical and politically acceptable." Most are just band-aid solutions that I consider minimalist and incremental. As the Kaiser Family Foundation, a highly reputable source of health policy analysis, bluntly put it recently (in a little noticed 2005 study), "none of the usual policy options raised in health policy or political circles is likely to significantly close the gap between the growth of health spending and [national] income."[6] No one, in short, really knows in a pragmatic sense what to do with a problem that is both real and threatening. The public has heard about and experienced the cost problem, but they have heard little about the pessimism, almost despair, that has marked some of the most important studies of it.[7]

With health care reform in general, there are many novel ideas in the air, often accompanied by a strategy to implement them. But specifically for the management of technology, most general proposals do not encompass an implementation strategy. Why is that? That is the question I wish to deal with in this volume: trying to understand why the control of technology intimidates politicians and health care administrators alike; why technology has unusually deep roots in American culture and commerce; and why the tried and effective means of controlling technology in Europe have such difficulty gaining acceptance here. Then I want to offer some concrete strategies for managing technology, propose some benchmarks for success in doing so, and try to show that nothing less than a cultural revolution in our thinking about progress, technology, death and aging will suffice to do the job.

I will use the Medicare program as my point of departure for a variety of reasons. With the advent of retirement looming for the baby boom generation, the weight of an aging society on health care will soon be felt with its full force; and that pressure will be set within a health care system already in deep trouble. As a government-financed program, Medicare can rightly be described as universal health care for the elderly. It thus offers a test case of managing that kind of system in the United States, one that will be useful if a universal government-regulated system ever emerges.

But I stress that Medicare is *only* my point of departure, and I will move in and out of Medicare cost considerations and those of a more general kind. Even without universal care, the present Medicare program is heavily influenced by American health care practices and policies. Medicare cannot be reformed in a cost-saving way without simultaneously changing that background dynamic. Medicare's important and ever-growing role in American health care means that the health care system cannot be reformed without drastically changing Medicare. The dilemma is a dynamic two-way street. The retirement of the baby boomers will be the great demographic event of the first half of the twenty-first century, just as the birth of that generation was the great demographic event of the last half of the twentieth century.

The analysis will proceed on two levels. One of these will be an examination of the available data and information on the impact of technology on health care costs, the nature of that impact, and the proposed and actual means of attempting to cope with them. I will argue that many of the most discussed ways of managing technology costs are minimalist and utterly insufficient to do much good. I will also argue that, like it or not, we will have to look toward European health care systems for effective means of dealing with costs—or fashion a compromise situation meant to bring together European and American values in some politically acceptable way. Not an easy exercise.

The other level is that of culture and politics. I do not believe we can effectively cope with the practical managerial, organizational, and policy issues without attempting to change many underlying cultural, social, and ethical premises. We have a culture addicted to the idea of unlimited progress and to the technological innovation that is its natural child. In its present form, this is an unsustainable value. There must be limits. American health care is radically American: individualistic, scientifically ambitious, market intoxicated, suspicious of government, and profit-driven. I put changing those values within health care in the class of a cultural revolution dedicated to finding and implementing a new set of foundational values.

The medical model that needs change encompasses a combination of Manichean and utopian values: that suffering of any kind, but mainly biological suffering, is an inherent evil; that death is intrinsically wrong and should be the main enemy of medicine; that the antiageism movement of recent decades is de facto acting as if old age were a biological anachronism, to be transcended even if not quite eliminated; and that endless medical progress should be pursued. There is, many seem to believe, no such thing as enough good health. Those are understandable values, the Enlightenment played out in medicine. They have become, however, the wrong ones to undergird health care systems and the practice of a medicine that aims for equitable access, a good balance between health and other social needs, and that are affordable, sustainable in the long run, and accessible to all.

Although there seems at first no direct connection discernible between them, it is remarkable that global warming is now, finally, being taken seriously in the United States; and that there is, simultaneously, a fresh push for serious health reform. In both cases, some deeply seated values must be changed, amounting in the end to fundamental alterations in our way of life. The drive for progress and constantly growing prosperity in the industrial order is behind the emergence of global warming; and an analogous drive has created the cost crisis in health care. In both cases, technology occupies a central place. In each instance, a basic question is whether we should be prepared to sacrifice some of the present and future benefits of science and technology, which have created the parallel dangers, or look to them for new initiatives to rescue us from the unwanted complications they have created.

The problems of Medicare ought to force us to think about the war against death, aging as a part of life, the place the elderly should have in our common life, obligations between young and old for their mutual flourishing, and what kind of resources— medical, social, and financial— should be devoted to health care in general and as well as to elder welfare. In particular, the American health care system as a whole raises an even wider range of basic questions. What is most important in health care? Staving off death and lengthening our life expectancy? Curing all the lethal and dread diseases? Helping us to cope with pain, suffering, and disability even if they do not kill us? Is quality of life more important than length of life? How do we balance the claims of different age groups? Those are the ultimate questions in thinking about health care but ones rarely confronted in the political debate about reform. Questions of that kind make politicians nervous, and thus they remain outside the scope of conventional economic and policy analysis. I will try to show these questions cannot be avoided.

Chapters 1–5 provide an analysis of the cost problem for Medicare and the underlying health care system. Their principal aim is to show that the cost problem is serious and urgent and that efforts to address it are marked by ambivalence and hesitation, in great part out of fear that technological innovation could be stifled. How can we control, much less cut back on, a medical technology that has had so many historical benefits and can bring so many more in the future? We can achieve this only if we are willing to take tough steps and admit that medical technology's economic harms can often exceed its benefits. The public will not strongly object to cutting physician fees or hospital reimbursements (although they may indirectly feel the consequences), but any thought of controlling or reducing the use of technology will seem to be much more direct and personal. I also consider the arguments for competition as a basic means for controlling costs as well as examine the relationship of American medicine and the medical industry.

Chapters 6, 7, and 8 present a set of revised values on which to base health care reform. These values will encompass a rejection of the reigning model of limitless medical progress and technological innovation, the use of the different stages of life, from childhood through old age, as a foundation for health policy, and setting health care priorities on the basis of the statistically most likely needs that people will have over their lifetime. I will offer a strong, perhaps utopian, plan and a less extreme parallel set of reforms, hoping that my more lofty proposals might someday prevail but, more realistically, propose a possibly more palatable menu of options, but one that would push us farther along. I will make clear my own bias toward the more radical possibilities but try to be plausible with the compromise possibilities.

The improvement of health, the relief of suffering, and the forestalling of death are as open-ended as the exploration of outer space. In each case, the possibilities are endless: no matter how far we go, there is always further we could travel. If we all lived an average of 150 years, the offices of the doctors would still be full, patients would still be looking to have their diseases cured, their pain and suffering relieved. Learning how to manage medical technology, which constantly extends the frontiers of medicine but requires economic limits, will be a vital first step toward a sustainable health care system.

CHAPTER 1

MEDICARE ON THE ROPES

F ew government programs have been as popular as Medicare. Its reputation is a triumph in a country prone to think poorly of government and of the regulations, waste, and bureaucracy widely believed to be its bastard child. It is hardly a perfect program, yet it has endured for over 45 years, and, save for some strong market advocates, only a few propose that it should be significantly changed, much less abolished.

Yet along with American health care more generally, Medicare is coming into increasingly difficult, even threatening, times. The health care system, of which Medicare is a key part, is beset by an excessive rate of cost escalation (now about 7% a year). Although it has controlled costs better than the private sector (a 1%–2% annual advantage), Medicare's costs are rising as well. And to create a twin threat, those costs are rising just as millions of the baby boom generation are moving into their retirement years. Medicare's budget is projected to climb from its present $427 billion in 2007 to $884 billion in 2017.[1] A Fidelity Investments study concluded that a 65-year-old couple retiring in 2008 would need $225,000 in savings to cover medical costs in retirement, encompassing co-payments and deductibles, Medicare-premiums, and out-of-pocket prescription costs.[2]

Although Medicare is my point of departure, its vitality (not necessarily its mere survival) is heavily dependent upon the fate of American health care more generally. The future of both will depend upon their mutual capacity to control costs. An important element in managing the cost escalation problem will depend upon the American willingness to rein in its long-stranding commitment to unlimited medical progress and technological innovation as its cherished outcome. I use the word "willingness" to indicate the importance of a change of both will and outlook, requiring a concerted moral and social drive in a fresh direction. The word "ability" is meant to underscore the difficulty, in the face of many competing interests, economic and cultural, to effect what even the most concerted drive for reform seeks. As Marilyn Moon, a long-time analyst of Medicare, put it: "the patterns of spending growth are very similar to and often below those of private insurance ... [But] Medicare (and Medicaid) cannot be successful in holding down costs over the long run if healthcare spending in general is escalating. ... Medicare's size also increases the responsibility to the overall financial health of the healthcare system."[3]

MEDICARE'S DILEMMA: MORE MONEY OR LESS?

For all of its popularity, Medicare has always had problems and critics. Its benefit structure rewards the use of technologies and those physicians who deploy them. It is heavily focused on acute care medicine, which it generously covers. It does not provide anywhere near decent coverage for prevention, talking with patients, and good primary care. As the geriatrician Christine K. Cassel has emphasized, it fails to provide coordinated treatment management and to address "the growing importance of self-care, chronic care, and low tech approaches to support quality of care and to reduce suffering."[4] Another important geriatrician, Muriel Gillick, has pointed out that "if Medicare is a good program for robust elders, it is profoundly inadequate for people who are frail or nearing the end of life."[5] If care of the chronically ill is a weak point, there is also persistent underfunding of Medicare's administrative structure. Attempts to move Medicare as an agency from one that pays the bills to an active manager of improved health have been thwarted by its skimpy staff and various other limitations built into the program.[6]

Medicare has always faced an obvious dilemma: to fulfill its original promise, it needs more money to improve administratively as a federal agency and to strengthen the quality and scope of its coverage, all the while trying to hold spending down. Higher quality and lower costs, that win/win combination, are not inconceivable, but at times look like the health care version of squaring the circle.

If Medicare faces a range of problems now, it is remarkable that it came into existence at all. In the years prior to its 1965 passage, it faced considerable resistance in Congress, lobbied against by the American Medical Association and many business groups. As the political scientist Jonathan Oberlander succinctly summed up the situation: "During the 1950s and early 1960s, Medicare emerged as a polarizing issue in American politics. Its legislative history bore the markings of a deeply ideological and partisan debate that reflected persistent divisions over the failed national health insurance proposals of the Truman administration."[7] All that changed rapidly with the 1964 elections and the advent of liberal democratic majorities in the House and Senate. When Medicare was launched by Congress, it was met by great public acclaim. If for many it was seen as prelude to universal health care, which did not happen, the program was itself a remarkable piece of legislation, overcoming deeply entrenched political opposition.

Once underway, Medicare enjoyed a long era, from 1965 to 1994, of bipartisan support and consensus, encouraged in great part by its popularity. From time to time the program had to cope with budgetary pressures to limit expenditures, on one hand, and political pressures to improve its benefits, on the other. The latter pressures were particularly strong because of gaps in the program (e.g., an absence of drug coverage) but also because of public opinion that pressed for benefit expansion, especially with the political force of elderly interest groups behind it.

A 1986 poll showed that 80% of the public supported Medicare expansion, even wanting more long-term care (covered by Medicaid). Nor was that just an expression of hope. The polls also overwhelmingly showed that the public was willing to accept a tax increase to bring the improvements about.[8] Even so, program benefits remained more or less unchanged over the years. Yet from the start, Congress was worried about the cost of Medicare, which soon came to seem out of control to many of its members. Unable to stop the cost increases of the program, cost containment as a priority triumphed over program improvement. One result was the development of private Medigap insurance, most of it limited to coverage of co-payments and deductibles, an initiative that relieved Congress of some of the pressure to improve benefits.

Over time, however, out-of-pocket per annum payments by the elderly for their health care increased and are now over $5000 on average and as high as $9000–10,000 for some. By 2003, the median Medicare beneficiary was spending 15.5% of income on health care, up from 11.9% in 1997. The government's share of Medicare beneficiary costs is about 60% coverage, although 75–80% is the rough standard of adequacy for private sector coverage.[9] Even so, Medicare has remained remarkably popular. It may well be that the security it offers more than makes up for its many shortcomings.

By the mid-1990s, the era of consensus was over. The earlier era was based on acceptance of the idea that Medicare would be a single-payer program resting on liberal principles, notably the conviction that it should be a social insurance program applicable to all the elderly, rich or poor, and highly resistant to means testing. The 1994 elections, with Republicans capturing both houses of Congress, reintroduced many of the partisan and ideological battles that had marked the era just before the introduction of Medicare. The drive to privatize the program took its first strong steps in the late 1990s, and it was combined with efforts to cut taxes and to reduce Medicare expenditures.

As it turned out, Medicare survived those years more or less intact. If liberal Democrats over the years could not improve Medicare benefits, a single-minded Republican and conservative assault could not seriously cut them. Why not? The best answer seems to be a potent combination of the popularity of the program, a wide range of financial and other interests favoring the status quo, and a pervasive nervousness about tampering with the program. "Both Democrats and Republicans know," David A. Hyman has written, "they are unelectable if they speak candidly about the economic problems facing Medicare. Republicans accordingly package their reform proposals as attempts to 'modernize' the Medicare benefit package and offer beneficiaries more options. Democrats focus their efforts on price caps and prayer."[10] That is a colorful exaggeration but on target. Christine Cassel makes a related, but no less frustrated, point: "Reformers are looking more toward incrementally adjusting benefits and deductibles, like a commercial insurer, than toward organizing to fulfill a vital public mandate."[11]

IS THERE A MEDICARE CRISIS?

As the global warming debate constantly reminds us, there is hardly any alleged social, political, or environmental threat that does not have its contrarians. However strong the general consensus of coming dangers, there are those who either question them, downplay them, or deny them altogether. The future of Medicare is no exception. Alternatively, the threat may be conceded, but pessimism rejected: with a little ingenuity and a strong will, solutions can be found. Pious hope can replace over-wrought pessimism.

It is not at all difficult to be a contrarian. Long-term financial and demographic projections are always uncertain. Who foresaw the baby boom generation coming in the 1930s? Medical cures and break-throughs, of great importance in charting future costs, cannot be pre-dicted: think of the discoveries of penicillin as well as other antibiotics and antivirals, radically reducing deaths from infectious disease. Or, for that matter, recall that just as infectious disease seemed by the 1970s to be conquered, antibiotic resistance and AIDS emerged, now threatening to overturn the earlier medical victories. And of course, Medicare itself has over its history faced many alleged budgetary "crises" but has man-aged to muddle through, sometimes stronger, sometimes weaker.

There are a number of reasons now to take the problem of credibility with particular seriousness. There is the clearly visible 7% annual cost increase with no end in sight. And the baby boom generation is, so to speak, already in the pipeline, waiting to retire, and to start flowing at a rapid and increasing rate after 2010, with horrendous projections by 2020 and even worse ones by 2030. Michael Leavitt, Secretary of the Department of Health and Human Services at the end of the Bush ad-ministration, was no contrarian. In an address in April 2008 he bluntly said that "Medicare is drifting toward disaster."[12] "It troubles me," he added, "that this matter is not receiving more attention in the presiden-tial candidates' discussion."

If Medicare faces a dire situation in the next 10 years or so, then steps must be taken now to drastically reform the program. It will be too late then—or too late to put in place anything but last-minute draconian stop gaps. But hardly anything is harder in politics and social policy than to take present steps to avert future dangers, and all the more if the needed reforms themselves will be demanding, even painful. Not much contrarian skepticism or opposition, even if it is a tiny minority voice, is needed to make the solution of present problems, not future ones, the default option. "Delay," the economist Peter Heller has written, "ex-poses societies to far greater risks than if the inevitable adjustment has been anticipated and implemented much earlier. . . . so governments . . . need to take much more explicit account in the near term of the potential fiscal consequences of long-term developments, despite the uncertainties that surround them."[13]

Moreover, if the argument of this book is plausible—that nothing less than a rethinking of some fundamental values is needed—then a strong consensus indeed will be necessary to deflect attention away from the organizational and management schemes that presently dominate mainline American reform efforts: just make the system work better. That kind of approach is a dead end, but a pursuit of such efforts can be likened to one of the endemic problems of end-of-life care, that of embracing hope and unlikely treatments and of refusing to grant the obvious fact that the patient is dying. Do not give up: provide one more round of chemotherapy. Do not give up: provide one more effort toward improving the efficiency and cutting waste in the health care system.

THE PESSIMISM OF THE MEDICARE TRUSTEES

The most pessimistic judgments on Medicare's financial problems have always come from the Trustees of its Trust Fund. Because the program still exists over 40 years later, it is not hard to become wary of, even jaded by, the traditional hand-wringing of its Trustees. For much of its history, the Medicare Trust Fund has projected a long-term deficit. At some future point, the Trustees have repeatedly said, its expenses will outrun its income (from payroll taxes in the case of hospital care, part A). But it has presented a peculiar kind of problem: the projected date of bankruptcy has fluctuated over the years, always pushed back to a later date. In 1966, the estimated date of exhaustion was 1990, or 24 years. In 1986, the exhaustion date was 1997, 11 years to go. By 2006 the date moved to 2024, or 18 years. Now it is down to ten years. The source of the fluctuation has been a mixture of higher and lower government revenue, changing medical costs, and a regular dose of anxiety "crisis" politics designed to avert fiscal threats. The fact that Medicare has continued despite the dire forecasts is at least one reason why some commentators expect that it will continue doing so: whatever its problems, Congress will not allow Medicare to go under.

Once again the language of crisis is being used, but this time with greater urgency than in the past and repeating other recent warnings. The 2008 report of the Board of Trustees of the Federal Hospital Insurance Fund (Part A) said that "HI [hospital insurance] tax income began falling short of HI expenditures in 2004 and is projected to do so in all future years . . . and fund assets are projected to be exhausted in 2019. . . . Consideration of . . . reforms should occur in the relatively near future . . . We believe that prompt, effective, and decisive action is necessary to address these challenges."[14] Medicare expenditures represented 2.7% of GDP in 2005, grew to 3.2% in 2006, and are projected to rise to 7.3% in 2035.[15]

Echoing the Trustee anxieties, the Congressional Budget Office (CBO) has noted that, along with an increase in the proportion of GDP spent on Medicare, the number of beneficiaries has increased from 20 million in 1970 to 41 million by 2003, with an increase as well in their average age. Most notably, costs per enrollee grew at a rate 3% faster than per capita GDP.[16] Another federal agency, the Congressional Research Office (CRS), combining Medicare and Medicaid projections, forecasts a rise from 4% of GDP today to 12% of GDP in 2030 to a staggering 21% in 2050. It notes that "relatively small tax increases or benefit reductions could return Social Security to long-run solvency."[17] But it could offer no silver lining for Medicare and Medicaid: "to finance projected increases in spending . . . would require tax increases of an unprecedented magnitude. . . . Under current policy, future generations will be made worse off by higher taxes or lower benefits."[18]

To highlight this point further, the CRS notes that, short of serious reform, health care deficits will grow from 6.1% to 12.3% of the GDP by 2030 and from 14.3% to 35% in 2050—and adds that the United States has never had a peacetime deficit greater than 6%.[19] The economic effects of even lower projections would do severe economic damage to the country, pushing it far beyond its borrowing and financing capacities. Moreover, with current policies unchanged, the Medicare Trust Fund will lack necessary resources well before the Fund is exhausted. Tax revenue is neither projected to rise nor costs projected to fall in any way sufficient to keep up with program spending.

An important provision of the Medicare legislation is meant to control the costs of Part A, hospital insurance. If general revenues to support the program (as distinguished from payroll taxes) are projected to exceed more than 45% of total income for 2 years within the next 7 years, then the president is required to propose changes to keep it below that level. In 2007, that triggering point was reached. President Bush, as required by law, then proposed cuts to stay below the 45% level. He proposed a 12.8% reduction in spending for Medicare, as well as research cuts, less money for teaching hospitals, and cuts in the budget of the Centers for Disease Control and Prevention.

His proposals evoked howls of protest, ranging from "deeply troubling" to a "disastrous impact." Senator Edward Kennedy said that Congress could simply do what it had done previously, giving those programs more money than suggested by the president. Not incidentally, Congress canceled the 10% physician reimbursement reduction plan, which it has regularly done over the years. In short, despite the Medicare Trustees' report, and its call for immediate action, or the legal requirement that the president specify cuts, he got nothing but blame; and no legislator suggested any alternative cuts to those proposed by the president. Congress aggressively went the other way, adding $20 billion in new benefits. One could hardly ask for a more telling example of Congress's unwillingness to cut costs, however much the need to do so has been by now well recognized. Even taking into account President Bush's unpopularity, I have no doubt that a Democratic president would have received a similar response, whatever the proposed cuts.

A long-standing maxim is that unsustainable growth rates will not be sustained. One way or another, they will be dealt with. Medicare will not be an exception; it cannot be. Or perhaps that assertion should be qualified. It is imaginable, although not too plausible, that the present medical struggle against suffering, aging, and death could ever more deeply embrace the language and paradigm of war, requiring all sorts of financial and social risks to vanquish the enemy. There are already some voices contending that the pursuit of health is a fine and popular enterprise and that, in the end, it does not matter how much of our GDP goes to health care. The transformation of old age, moreover, which many seek, goes hand-in-hand with that perspective. What better way to spend money? Although it might not stop reform efforts, that attitude might well enervate the will to carry them out, filling the room with a sweet-smelling, seductive odor, a kind of utopian carbon monoxide, present but not quite visible.

In the meantime, there are many possible ways of financially supporting Medicare, some seriously pursued, others still in the realm of speculation and theory. These can conveniently be classified into two categories: (1) changes in the financing and regulation of the present government-dominated program, but with no change in its underlying philosophy; and (2) changes in the relationship between government and the private sector, and particularly a movement toward greater privatization of the program, and thus a change in its philosophy.

MEDICARE REGULATORY AND FINANCING REFORM

Over the years, four principal modes of financial reform have been proposed for Medicare: the addition of general revenue funds, an increase in payroll taxes, reduction of benefits or increased cost-sharing, and a whittling away of payments to doctors and hospitals. None of these strategies would change the underlying original philosophy of the program.

THE USE OF GENERAL REVENUE FUNDS

Medicare is now financed from payroll taxes. In the face of trust fund shortfalls, additional funds could be made available by drawing on general federal tax revenues. Over the years, there has been persistent political resistance to that solution. Worries about maintaining the fiscal discipline of the program, a wish to obscure its true costs, and a desire to keep it as a self-financing program are some of the reasons for that resistance. It does not now seem to have any political support, but that could change.[20] Other financing methods are conceivable: taxation of motor car fuel and/or of alcohol and cigarettes, a tax on Medicare benefits, or a value-added-type tax (VAT) on consumption.[21]

INCREASING THE PAYROLL TAX

There has for many years been resistance to an increase in the rate of payroll taxation, now set at 1.45% of taxable salary. Yet it may well be that the long resistance to an increase has come not from the public, which (according to public opinion surveys) has long been open to an increase, but from Congress. A concern about intergenerational equity, placing an increased burden upon the working young to support the elderly has been suggested as a strong reason for this resistance. "The political limit on Medicare payroll taxes," Jonathan Oberlander has observed, "has been less a function of public opinion than of elite preferences."[22]

Increasing Beneficiary Costs

Cost-sharing through co-payments or deductibles on the part of Medicare beneficiaries has been on the increase of late and rose sharply in 2007. Most notably, those with a high income will pay considerably more than others for Medicare Part B, covering physician care, and thus was introduced means testing, a move long resisted by Medicare advocates but supported by public opinion surveys. Despite considerable discussion of late about an increase in the age of eligibility for Medicare coverage, any change has yet to be enacted (unlike Social Security, which will raise the age of eligibility to 67 in 2027). The CBO, however, has pointed out that even if the age of eligibility for Medicare were raised to 67 by 2027 (to coincide with the scheduled Social Security increase), it would lower health care costs by only 4%. A move to the age of 70 would decrease enrollment by 18%, but reduce costs by only 9%. Its report then adds that "even that relatively dramatic policy change would do little to address the long-range fiscal challenge facing Medicare."[23]

Lowering Payments to Health Care Providers

Perhaps because they attract the least public attention, lowering the reimbursements to hospitals and doctors has been a favorite cost-control tactic over the years. Both groups protest vigorously, however, and, often enough, their complaints win out, and these cuts are rescinded. Just how far this strategy can go is unclear. The CBO again strikes a pessimistic note: "Because Medicare limits the amount that providers may charge enrollees over and above the program's payment rates, if providers could not charge enough to cover the costs of providing a service, this policy could restrict Medicare patients' access to care." [24] As the proportion of the elderly in the population begins to grow rapidly, Medicare patients will have to remain financially attractive to physicians if they are to receive good care.

Public Opinion

Although there is not now, and probably never will be, a good correlation between public opinion and the way Congress acts and legislates, public opinion polls suggest why it is hesitant to make any great Medicare changes. The most persistent theme over the years in the surveys is that the program is very popular, with 70–80% of the population favorable toward it. "The majority of Americans support the underlying principles of Medicare," one public opinion study found, "as a public program, a basic right, and a 'social contract.'"[25] Yet, while the public strongly supports the program as a government, not private, program, it also shows a willingness to take some personal responsibility for health care costs. A majority of citizens have little confidence that future benefits will be equal to present benefits, just as a majority also believe the program faces major troubles—and supports in a vague way an increase for Medicare in the federal budget.[26]

But a recognition of the problem does not readily translate into support of specific means to control Medicare's budget. About the only reform with any consistent support over the years has been that of imposing a higher tax rate on the affluent; and that has now happened (although it will provide a small relief only, less than 1% of the annual Medicare budget). Politicians and legislators surely know that the public considers the problems of Medicare to be serious. They also know that there is no strong public mandate to reform the program in ways that will keep it solvent and sustainable.

A *Wall Street Journal*/Harris poll taken just prior to the November 2006 congressional elections found that, although 42% of those polled saw the problem of the uninsured as of top importance, Medicare reform was of high importance to only 28%.[27] Hardly less disturbing, the public poorly understands how the Medicare program itself works. Fraud and waste have for many years mistakenly been identified as the main culprits pushing up costs, just as many people do not understand that Medicare does not pay for long-term nursing care (which is Medicaid's responsibility). The need for public and media education is strong, but there are few available funds to carry out that task.[28] At the least, the public needs to understand that, without reform, the Medicare cash deficit will move from the present small annual deficits to close to $100 billion by 2020 and close to $300 billion by 2035. The public should also know that, one way or the other, there will doubtless be reform. The public likes the current program too much for Congress to abandon it. The serious question then becomes: will the reforms, or just change, come much too late, more like a defeated army in rout, marked by the chaos of sharp benefit cuts and increased co-payments and deductibles?

The previous paragraph was written in 2007, and I decided to let it stand as an indication of how sharply public opinion has changed between then and mid-2008. A 2008 Kaiser Family Foundation election tracking poll noted that in June of 2007 only 13% of those surveyed cited the economy as the main issue they would like to see the presidential candidates talk about. By April of 2008, that figure had jumped to 49%. Where Iraq was the main issue in March of 2007, it came second to the economy in April of 2008. Health care came in third behind the economy and Iraq in March of 2007, with 27% only of those polled wanting the candidates to discuss it, and by April 2008 had declined to 23%.[29]

CONTROLLING MEDICARE COSTS

Although a major focus in considering Medicare's bleak future has been on either raising taxes or cutting benefits or both—and probably in draconian ways—another possibility is to better control the costs of the program. Given that those costs will inevitably rise as the number of beneficiaries grows, it is the combination of that rise together with a simultaneous increase in technology-driven costs that poses the greatest hazard. And if history proves any guide, these technology gains fuel a steady raising of the psychological and social baseline of what counts as "acceptable medical care" and, thus, of public demand. It is not just that the baby boomers will cost more. There are good reasons to believe they will expect more, which of course is an important reason they will cost more—a self-perpetuating circle.

An important and detailed study of Medicare's efforts over the years, published by the AARP Public Policy Institute in 2008, shows a mixture of successes and failures. Its most notable successes have been the superiority of Medicare over the private sector in holding down annual cost increases, and its episode-based prospective payment system in restraining hospital cost increases. The latter is of particular importance because around 32% of Medicare costs are in hospital care, the most important component of its expenditures. Its failures (which will be discussed at various points later in this book) include a failure to hold down physician fee-for-service costs (successful for much of the 1990s but rising again after 2000), and its inability to persuade Congress to allow it to use more evidence-based and cost-effectiveness data in its coverage decisions. "Although there have been some moves in that direction," the study notes, "altering the bases for making coverage decisions faces formidable obstacles, both political and technological, in the face of concerns about limiting beneficiary access to cutting-edge technology." That last item will be a recurrent theme in the pages that follow.

For at least 38 years now, since the Nixon administration, there has been a widespread belief, almost a certainty in some quarters, that medical research and the technological innovation that flows from it will eventually reduce the cost of health care. For many years this conviction made use of the writings of the late Lewis Thomas, famous for pointing out that much medical technology (this was during the 1960s and 1970s) is a half-way technology, keeping people alive but not curing them.[30] Research, he was convinced, would produce cures and thus make the technology unnecessary. With the chronic diseases of the elderly, this has not happened. Heart disease, cancer, and respiratory diseases account for well over half of all deaths. The cost of treating the five most costly conditions increased from $227 billion in 2000 to $311 billion in 2004, a 37% increase.[31] The same era saw the introduction of the idea of a compression of morbidity, which would see a reduction in lifetime illness followed by a quick, inexpensive death after a long life.[32] Hardly less common was an expectation that increased medical research would lead to treatments and cures that would eventually cut costs. For all the chronic optimism, that has not happened. As the CBO put it, "examples of new treatments for which long-term savings have been demonstrated are few."[33] The idea that more research will reduce health care costs is a myth. It raises them. Will that always prove true? If history is our tutor, you may count on it.

Perhaps the most pervasive optimism has come from the faith that, given the waste and inefficiency in American health care, surely remediable, costs could be controlled: "cut the fat" and improve inefficiency has been the cry. In the mid-1990s another expected remedy, Health Maintenance Organizations (HMOs), did in fact lead to a short-term flattening of cost increase, but public and professional resistance to exactly those features necessary for cost control proved to be exceedingly unpopular with physicians and patients; the success was short-lived.

With the possible exception of the compression of morbidity, which has to some extent happened, none of the other proposed panaceas has worked. That fact, as we shall see, has not stopped the use of oft-repeated arguments in their favor. Hope continues to triumph over history and failed efforts. The reasons for failure are not hard to locate. There has been a steady stream of new and usually expensive technologies, a wider range of medical pathologies that can be treated with them, and—when the cost of various technologies comes down—an increase in the number of those who use them. Imaging devices—CT scans, PET scans, and MRIs—have all seen some decline in costs per individual case but have also experienced a massive expansion of users. And there has been continued waste and inefficiency, the chronic illness of a chaotic, fragmented health care system. As for the impact of research, one calculation has shown that even if cancer, diabetes, and heart disease were eliminated, the savings in elder health care costs would, by 2020 and beyond, lead to a savings of only 10% in the overall costs.[34] Curing disease—fairly rare these days with the major diseases—does not cure death. It just moves it to some other lethal condition, and the cost thereby moves with it.

THE END OF OPTIMISM

The chronic optimism about research may now be on the wane, or at least tempered. Forty years of failure to control costs has been sobering. The Harvard economist David Cutler has become well known for his efforts to show that much of the high cost of research and of health care, although it does indeed drive up costs is "worth it." The social and economic benefits of healthier populations and longer lives are as fine a return on investment as any other way of spending money. Yet when it comes to elder costs, he concedes, that return may be less so. Medical spending has gone up at a rate of 10% a year for the past 40 years.[35] "The increase in life expectancy beginning at 65 years of age showed the incremental cost of an additional year of life rose from $46,800 in the 1970s to $145,000 in the 1990s. . . . If this trend continues in the elderly, the cost-effectiveness of medical care will continue to decrease at older ages."[36] To put that judgment more bluntly: we are achieving ever higher costs for ever smaller health gains.

Although it is hard to find evidence that the 40-year mantra of increased efficiency and reduction of waste will help control costs has borne any significant fruit, it remains strong, perhaps because it would allow a continuation of the status quo of such root values as technological innovation. The work of John Wennberg at Dartmouth over the years has focused on practice and treatment variations in different regions of the country, hospital usage, and in end-of-life care. He and his colleagues have estimated that 20% of Medicare expenditures are spent for "health care with no measurable survival benefit."[37] But even if those variations could be managed better, and no way has been found to do that, even a 20% cut in expenditures would not go far in lowering the massive escalations ahead.

As Dana P. Goldman, Director of the RAND Program on Health Economics, has emphasized, "ultimately, society faces its greatest spending risk not from demographic and health trends, but rather from health technologies."[38] He and his colleagues at Rand—developed as part of a Future Elderly Model (FEM) analysis— have devised a number of studies whose results are exceedingly pessimistic about controlling technology-driven costs. In particular, they (along with others) have shown that one long-cherished hope is not turning out as expected: that decreasing disability among the elderly will necessarily lead to decreasing costs. On the contrary, because those elderly without serious disabilities are more likely to live longer than those with them, the lifetime costs will be about the same (including the extended period of Social Security and long-term care coverage).[39] Rising rates of obesity, meanwhile, will make matters worse. Medicare is projected to spend 30% more on obese patients than on others.[40] As for the likelihood that new cancer cures and treatments will reduce costs, "no scenario [of future medical progress] holds major promise for guaranteeing the future financial health of Medicare."[41]

David Cutler, summing up the findings of the various studies included in the special *Health Affairs* issue reporting the findings of the FEM work, said that "the papers here could well lead to despair. . . . To some extent, dire predictions about Medicare are unavoidable. . . . one would need to cut medical spending for the elderly in 2050 more than in half to balance spending with revenue forecasts. No one has a way to do that."[42] Even so, Cutler seems compelled to find some hope. Medicare spending, he concludes, will go up, "but there is enormous potential for cost savings as well, which we have the capacity to realize. One can be an optimist even when the storm clouds are gathering." Even economists can play Pollyanna.

Uncomfortably, the "potential for cost savings" has always been present and for many decades now. The historical track record of such hopes is abysmal. The health care inflation rate has fluctuated, to be sure, between 7% and 12%, but even the low end is no longer tolerable. Not only must individual inefficiencies be dealt with, which is hard enough, but to make a major budgetary difference, all or most of the cost-saving interventions must be simultaneously successful, a heavy burden for a system that has barely succeeded in eliminating any major inefficiencies over many decades. There is no reason to expect Cutler's wish list will fare better than its myriad predecessors, much less as a group.

Although at the end of her fine book, *Medicare Matters*, Christine Cassel argues for the "inevitability of rationing" in the Medicare program, she also says early on (in a somewhat contradictory way) that "rationing appears unjustifiable when there are abundant opportunities to economize by improving efficiency and effectiveness in the health care system."[43] That kind of argument has been made for years as well, but if getting rid of inefficiency is a necessary precondition of rationing, that condition has not now, and may never, be fully met. I would contend, on the contrary, that rationing is necessary in order to provide serious incentives for improved efficiency. Only if there are clear denials of care because of cost will there be a strong impetus to do something about waste and inefficiency (many elements of which are clashes about the value of various diagnostic and therapeutic procedures). A procedure that saves only one life in a hundred is, for some, not wasteful but a respect for the value of life.

Mention was made earlier of the openings for contrarians that Medicare (and any other long-term projections on anything) offer. A prominent example is found in the writings of Joseph White, a professor of public policy at Case Western Reserve University. "The aging of the population does pose economic and budgetary challenges, but the contribution of health care costs to this equation is minor."[44] He arrives at that conclusion by noting what has been known for some time: that the contribution of aging per se to cost increases has to date not been an important cost driver. He does not mention the future, when the baby boomers retire, and the projection (cited above) of a doubling of elder costs between 2000 and 2030. He notes, almost in passing, that "technological progress" is a more important source of cost pressures. For some reason or other, he does not consider the possibility that such progress, applied to an ever larger portion of elderly, is what makes aging a serious problem; these are treated as utterly separate issues, which in reality they are not.

White rests his case, oddly enough, by saying there is "little ethical or financial reason to focus on reducing health care spending on the elderly," citing OECD studies of what various European countries are doing to deal with the aging problem: "eliminate early retirement schemes . . . raise standard retirement ages; increase childcare subsidies; eliminate tax discrimination against female participation; and enhance the role of part-time work."[45] But he fails to note the important differences between the European and American approach to aging societies. The European countries often deal with aging as a birthrate problem—hence the emphasis, entirely absent in the United States, of better financial support for working women in order that they will have greater economic freedom to have more children. At the same time, the Europeans are also aware that their own baby boom problem will pose cost issues as well, but the emphasis is different. In the United States by contrast, although it has not had a birthrate problem to date, there is a cost problem for the health care system as a whole and a projected critical one for the Medicare program.

THE MARKET MOVE

The reform proposals so far discussed assume that Medicare will remain a federally financed and managed social insurance plan, more or less as it was fashioned at the outset. The greatest challenge to that model comes from economic conservatives and Republican ideologies. Although there had been, prior to 1965, debates about a role for the market in the Medicare program, the Democrats of that era, riding high, fended off that approach. It was not until the 1994 Congressional elections, with the Republicans capturing both houses, that market advocacy and legislative success returned in a powerful way. Newt Gingrich and his conservative Contract with America made Medicare reform a top issue. The private sector was to be given a greater role in the program, reducing the government role: more patient choice, more provider competition, and less regulation.

That mid-1990s market move took some time to gain momentum, and it was the George W. Bush administration that, in 2003, achieved the greatest market triumph, pushing through a Republican Congress the Medicare Prescription Drug Improvement and Modernization Act

(MMA). The centerpiece of that Act was the creation of drug coverage as part of Medicare (part D), something long sought, particularly as pharmaceuticals gained an increasingly central place in health care. The negotiations over the act put the Democrats in a difficult position: they (and the public) had long wanted such coverage—but not necessarily at the cost of a substantial privatization of its coverage mechanisms.

The result of the Act was, in the words of a *Wall Street Journal* article, a classic compromise, "a Democratic benefit and a Republican delivery system."[46] Although the drug benefit program was the centerpiece of the MMA, the Act itself cut a wider market swath. It added medical savings accounts, government subsidies of private health plans to compete with Medicare's traditional fee-for-service coverage, a 28% tax exemption for corporations offering retiree drug benefits, and a reliance upon insurance companies and private health plans to manage the drug benefit. Most strikingly, the Act prohibited the government from negotiating lower drug prices for Medicare beneficiaries—a remarkable tactic for an Act that otherwise sought to embrace the market. All markets are equal, but some are more equal than others.

Many conservatives faulted the Act for its high cost calling it little more than one more "big government" program, which it is. "The conservative, free market base in America," the former Republican House majority leader Dick Armey said, "is rightly in revolt over this bill."[47] One cadre of market-oriented legislators had out-maneuvered another, still larger cadre. The former was accused during the Bush administration more than once of selling out conservative values, most notably a commitment to smaller government. But then no Republican administration has ever succeeded in achieving that goal.

If the MMA had some odd features for a "market" initiative—what could possibly be stranger than government subsidies as a jump-start strategy?—it must surely count as the most dramatic effort to date in that direction. It brought market ideas to the fore and then put some important market practices in place. And the drive for increased privatization of Medicare continues unabated, at least in terms of the zeal and energy of its advocates.

Most enacted and proposed market plans are speculative, lacking a track record at a national level by which to judge them. I stress the words "most" and "national," because there is some scattered evidence for and against their efficacy in narrower contexts (see chapter 4). What the market ideas have in common—consumer-directed health care—is the pursuit of greater patient choice, more provider competition, and by that strategy the control of costs. The working model is not drawn from health care practice and traditions but from business.

It is probably no accident that one of the leading American enthusiasts for consumer-directed health care (CDHC), Regina Herzlinger, is a faculty member at the Harvard Business School. Not only does she draw her model of health care directly from the business community, she also touts it with all the verve of a campaign worked up by the school's marketing department: "The U.S. health care system is in the midst of a ferocious war . . . a system controlled by the insurance companies or hospitals or government will kill us financially and medically . . . there is only one group that can prevent this damage: consumers—you and me—working together with our doctors."[48] It is probably no accident either that CDHC seems to be an excessively American idea, a combination of our distrust of government, our hyperindividualism, and our love of the market. Nonetheless, other countries are flirting with the idea in one form or another.

JUDGING MARKET PROPOSALS

If most of the market ideas are speculative in nature, it is pertinent to ask what criteria should be used in judging them and what evidence is necessary to evaluate them as sound and promising. I propose three levels of criteria. The first is the most fundamental: what should the baseline of comparative judgment be in choosing between a government-oriented and a market-oriented bias? My choice would be the present Medicare program, excluding (save for drug coverage) those market features introduced by the MMA. Although the program has many flaws, it is a highly popular program with its recipients, it has lower administrative costs than private health plans, and has controlled costs better than those plans. The fact that the life expectancy of Americans over 80 years is the highest in the world (close to 100% of whom are Medicare beneficiaries), is a striking note in its favor—and particularly when compared with the much lower life expectancy by international ranking for those under 65, covered mainly by private plans.[49] Hence, because it is already in place, is popular, and would be politically difficult to eliminate, it makes sense to use it as the baseline for comparison.

"If it ain't broke, don't fix it" is a time-honored and sensible principle. But because Medicare is broken in part, and always has been, an amended version may be offered: "if it is partially broke, but has many strengths, try to fix it before turning to the market." That standard would require market proposals to meet an important test: to show that they can do much *better* than the present program in order to justify a radical change in a program long in place with an instructive history, for good and bad.

The second criterion: what would the proposed market-oriented reforms do for the quality of care, affordable access to care, and to health outcomes? It is not altogether clear how to measure health outcomes of the present Medicare program comparatively, but the fact, as mentioned, that the United States leads the world in life expectancy beyond the age of 80, and the program is popular as well, surely gives it a leg up in any competition with the market. No doubt it could do better, but it is hardly evident that market moves could bring that outcome about.

The third criterion is that of controlling costs. Medicare lives under the cloud of future financial troubles, in great part because of the American health care system in which it is embedded and that heavily determines its costs. What likelihood is there that market practices would better cope with cost increase than a government-run system? And can those costs be managed in a way that could avoid simply shifting increases to the beneficiaries in an ultimately harmful way, particularly to low-income patients?

To try answering that question, I will simply describe present and proposed market moves and then provide some assessment of them as a group, reserving a full discussion of competition for chapter 4. I should note, however, that most of the market proposals for Medicare are also applicable to American health care more generally and can be found in both contexts.

MARKET STRATEGIES

As noted above, the MMA has already put some market elements into the present Medicare system. The Medicare Advantage program (previously Medicare+Choice), and called Medicare C, aims to allow beneficiaries to select a variety of private programs (HMOs, PPOs, and private fee-for-service plans). Although there are a variety of options under these plans, the aim is to package Medicare coverage, parts A and B, including in some cases drug coverage. Beginning in 2007, a medical savings account plan for Medicare was also established. Neither of these moves, even if widely accepted, promises any striking cost control results, and none is usually claimed, much less acclaimed.

The Federal Employees Health Benefits Program (FEHBP) is a federal program for government employees. Covering 75% of employee health care costs, it beneficiaries to choose from a number of health plans and to change those plans every year if they desire to do so. It has been proposed as a model for Medicare because of its relative simplicity of organization and its popularity with federal employees.[50] Beginning in 2010, the MMA provides for the development of a demonstration project to test its value. Yet by its dependence on private plans, it is held hostage to all of the problems of cost control experienced in the private sector and, with no power on the part of government to control their practices, much less costs (see chapter 4).

The FEHBP is a form of "defined contribution" and voucher plans. With employers mainly in mind, such plans provide for the provision of a set amount of money for employees to allow them to buy whatever health care they choose.[51] One proposed plan, pushed vigorously by Ezekiel Emanuel and Victor Fuchs in an article "Health Care Vouchers— A Proposal for Universal Coverage," calls for a government-provided voucher. For its participants, everyone eligible, it would "guarantee and pay for basic health services from a qualified insurance company or health plan."[52] Participants would also be free to buy additional services or amenities. Their plan would, like the MMA, combine "a Democratic benefit and a Republican delivery system" (although they do not phrase it that way). In the long run, the voucher plan would call for the elimination of employer-based insurance, the elimination of Medicaid and other means-tested programs, and a phasing out of Medicare. The projections for cost savings are as dramatic in their rhetoric as they are unsupported by any evidence to demonstrate this.

Beyond those market proposals for large-scale changes in Medicare and health care more generally are a number of smaller market moves that aim to privatize Medicare. The Medicare Advantage and Health Care Savings Account programs are the most prominent. The former aims to simplify Medicare coverage and to advance the use of HMOs and private health plans rather than traditional Medicare fee-for-service coverage. Health savings accounts are aimed at reducing the use of less expensive forms of health care but are buttressed by privately provided catastrophic care coverage. The Medicare Advantage program has existed for too short a time to assess its impact on costs, but the fact of a significant government subsidy makes a reduction implausible. It is flawed as a market tactic because it is subsidized by government and is more expensive than standard Medicare coverage. In 2008, its extra payments added $2.5 billion to Medicare costs beyond what they would have been under the traditional fee-for-service program.[53] Medical Savings Accounts provide some advantage for those with sufficient income to invest in them. Yet their chance of having any great cost benefit for the health care system is slight because over 80% of national health care costs are incurred by 20% of the population (and who need catastrophic care coverage), the savings that would come from hesitation to use the savings account money for lesser illnesses and cost-sharing would be minor.

Cutting through both government- and market-oriented plans and proposals are a number of other reform schemes, aimed at particular problems in general health care. They include the development and dissemination of information technology, evidence-based medicine (EBM) and clinical guidelines, improved quality of care, reduction of regional disparities, and more preventive medicine—and, as an old refrain—improved efficiency and a reduction of waste. On the whole, however, there seems to me to be a greater emphasis on such reforms among those who are government-oriented than among those with a market predilection. If my impression is correct, it may well be because all of such reforms, to be done well, would require a very active government role; private health care providers would not be as well positioned to pursue them.

RESPONSE TO PRIVATIZATION PRESSURES

I have found it exceedingly hard to work my way through the thicket of arguments and ripostes on the promise of market benefits in order to judge their validity. The arguments seem endless: large fights over uncertain data, promissory notes of claimed benefits but with no projected cost and benefit figures attached, and startling omissions on occasion of important considerations not considered. The underlying role played by ideologies and tacit value commitments is often hard to discern; a fog of facts, figures, and projections usually obscure them. Moreover, when there is some solidity in the proffered supportive data, the differences between them are usually only marginal.

I will single out two issues here that seem to me important, one of them ideological, the other technical. The ideological issue is that of the omission, save for the Medicare voucher-type proposals, of any attention at all to matters of equity and universality of case in the private plans. Those considerations are simply not present in most schemes to increase the role of private health care plans and a shifting of more costs to individuals. The market proposals reflect a single-minded drive to increase individual choice and to reduce the role of government, quite independently of their aggregate social impact and system-wide community implications.

The endemic technical omission is twofold: (1) a failure to calculate cost savings, with at least some projected (even if uncertain) figures to back up claims of cost-saving from competitive, administrative, and consumer-directed choices; and (2) its economic twin: the capacity of the market schemes to control costs over the long run. The most remarkable instance of those omissions is the Emanuel/Fuchs voucher plan, otherwise without even a hint of the kind of power its findings would have to *control* the technology behavior of the private plans that service the vouchers.

Beyond skepticism of that kind, private health care as an alternative to the present Medicare program is rejected from two directions. There are those who, like the distinguished Medicare experts, Marilyn Moon and Joseph White, believe that the present program needs major but not radical reform and that this can be done within the framework of the present program; and that such reform can on the whole take care of its economic and other threats. Their chosen strategy is incrementalism, positing a wide range of reform efforts gradually applied. A strong dose of privatization is neither needed nor desirable. It will not increase efficiency or significantly control costs. It is difficult, Moon shows, for "private plans to compete with Medicare on cost grounds. . . . Most private plans have not created new or innovative delivery systems that generate substantial savings while retaining consumer satisfaction."[54]

The other stream of criticism focuses on the threat to Medicare's most important historical feature, its character as a social insurance program aiming at equitable and affordable care for the elderly. That has been a principal source of its public acceptance and popularity. Privatization in whole or significant part would invite inequities, do harm to its poor and minority beneficiaries, and cut the heart out of its strongest claim, that rich and poor are treated alike.[55]

The European experience is relevant. Privatization of health care has moved forward in many European countries in recent years, in part as a way of dealing with costs but more importantly as a response to some public pressure for alternatives to the government systems. CDHC, in its milder incarnations, has gained a place. It mainly takes the form of private health insurance options parallel to the government systems, and to cost-sharing within those systems. It can be compulsory (Switzerland); substitutive, for those excluded from some aspects of the state system (The Netherlands, Belgium); complementary, for services excluded or not fully covered by the government program (Denmark, France, Italy); and supplementary, for an increased range of providers, faster access, and additional amenities (Spain, the UK, Sweden).[56]

A 2004 World Health Organization study had a blunt summary of its findings: "Evidence shows that private sources of health care funding are often regressive and present financial barriers to access. They contribute little to efforts to contain costs and may actually encourage cost inflation."[57] On cost containment, it noted that "private insurers have fewer incentives to contain costs [because] private health insurance is mainly paid for by individuals rather than employers."[58] It added that "publicly-funded systems are generally more successful in controlling cost inflation than systems that are mainly funded from private sources."[59] The study cites Canada and the UK because they "seem to be most successful in maintaining the lowest annual inflation rates."[60] The study should have added, however, that those systems have many problems because of their reliance on taxation, including waiting lists and shortage of doctors and nurses. The rising cost problem has been identified by the international Organization for Economic Cooperation and Cultural Development (OECD) as the main reason why the United States has a serious problem with elder care, despite otherwise being in a favorable position with its aging population. Many European countries, saddled with early retirement policies and lavish retirement benefits, have a different kind of elder problem.

Is there a Medicare crisis? I end this chapter with the same question with which it began. My short answer to the question is "yes," principally because, with Medicare as with the rest of American health care, the main problem is a steady cost escalation. And behind much of that escalation is technological innovation and the increased use of technology. With the expected flood of retiring baby boomers expected to start in 2010, the combination of rising costs and the rising number of elderly is a formidable threat. It is exceedingly difficult to find, in the most important Medicare studies, much sustained attention to the cost issue.

As if that alarm were not enough, the Kaiser Family Foundation, an exceedingly reputable, nonpartisan source of policy analysis, issued a report in 2006 that examined the gap between the annual growth of health care spending and national income. Can that cost increase be successfully stopped? Its answer: a decisive "no." To reach that answer, it surveyed a range of current cost control efforts: by *payers* (e.g., EBM, improved information technology, better management of high cost and chronically ill patients, reducing payment rates to providers); by the use of *consumer-directed* approaches (e.g. out-of-pocket payments, better information to allow more cost-conscious and informed choices, tax incentives); and *supply-side* strategies (e.g., electronic medical records, reduction of medical errors, rewarding efficiency and quality).[61]

Despite that wide range of efforts at every level of health care, the report concluded that "*Although many of these efforts may lead to efficiency and quality gains, none would appear to be of a scale to have any meaningful impact on the overall cost picture.*" [italics mine]. And it adds

> that the development and adoption of new medical technology . . . is responsible for a substantial portion of the growth in health expenditures. . . . To address the impact of medical technology on spending, policies would need to constrain the introduction and adoption of new medical products and services to a much greater extent than we do today.[62]

The economist Sherry Glied appends an exclamation point to that judgment when she adds, in restrained language, "the expenditure-increasing technological improvement is likely to continue in the future and does not appear highly responsive to policy changes."[63]

THE UNPLEASANT ROAD AHEAD

The contention of this chapter has been simple and blunt: there is no way that the Medicare program—or for that matter the health care system more generally—can remain sustainable, by which I mean affordable and equitable over the long run, unless it can control costs. So far, the track record in doing so has been strikingly weak, and most ideas for cost containment seem to me unlikely to make a great difference. The key to doing that is to better manage and rein in technological adoption and system utilization. Medicare has on average over the years done better than the private sector in that respect, but it is still far from a tolerable annual cost escalation, which would have to be in the 2–3% range, running parallel to the growth of GDP, to keep the program economically viable.

It is surely plausible and imaginable that taxation to support the program can in one way or another be raised, that benefits can be cut, and that co-payments and deductibles can be increased. But the hard question is twofold. How far could all that cost containment go before the program would, in effect, be gutted? That latter possibility is rarely mentioned, but is it not plausible if costs continue rising much faster than the GDP? Moreover, a thinning out has been the fate of more than one recent federal program, for instance, those of Pell grants for low-income college students, whose benefits have been radically cut, and the national welfare program, cut in the Clinton years, heightening eligibility standards and cutting benefits. As it happened with the latter, to be sure, many have argued that these measures have turned out well, forcing a large number of former recipients to try harder to find and keep jobs. It is difficult, however, to imagine that steadily rising out-of-pocket payments—forcing people to think twice and thrice about seeking medical care in the first place—would turn out to be a gain for health; and they would do little to deal with the costs of expensive critical care medicine, the current most important cost driver of the system.

Marilyn Moon has written that "if as a society we decide to support the Medicare program, we have the capability of doing so. . . . to serve one in every five Americans in 2025 will require substantial resources. Someone will have to pay more."[64] No doubt that is true, but unless costs are controlled the "more" could well turn out to be prohibitive— and that is just the path we are now on. Bruce Vladeck, a former Administrator of the Heath Care Financing Administration (the predecessor of the CMS), a no less acute observer of the Medicare program, has written that "What is clear is that the future of Medicare will be determined by political agendas far outside of Medicare itself. The struggle for the soul of Medicare is the struggle for the future of American society."[65] Given the value of unlimited progress behind American health care and Medicare, I would argue that rethinking the idea of technological progress is the key to that soul.

CHAPTER 2

TAMING THE BELOVED BEAST

MEDICAL TECHNOLOGY

I have likened medical technology to an unruly and untamed, but be-loved, beast: it saves and improves our lives with its undoubted power to diagnose and treat but, in its unrestrained lumbering about in the house of medicine, increasingly wreaks financial havoc. Is "havoc" too strong a word to use? Recall the figures presented in the previous chap-ter: a projected increase in the Medicare spending from $427 billion in 2006 to $884 billion in 2030. For the health care system as a whole, the figures move from $2.6 trillion in 2006 to $4.1 trillion in 2015.

That kind of increase is what we get from a projected long-term con-tinuation of a 7% annual cost escalation, close to half of which comes from technology spending. Recall as well those bleak Kaiser Family Foundation forecasts of the utter inadequacy of any present or even pro-posed policies to do much about the situation. For Medicare beneficiaries, the worst scenario is an eventual doubling of taxes to support the pro-gram (which their children will have to pay) or a cutting of benefits by half, or some combination of tax increase and benefit decimation. For everyone else, the situation will be a comparable mess.

Apart from those contrarians who minimize the problem, even those who recognize it focus almost exclusively on various cost control tactics rather than telling us what, ultimately, we should be aiming for. But it would be helpful to have a target end-point, one that (even subject to many qualifications) could tell us where we should be heading and what would be significant benchmarks along the way. From there one can move toward devising the means necessary to reach that point

To begin this exercise, some questions must be answered. How much money should be spent on health care, and what counts as "too much?"

What is a reasonably acceptable guideline in determining what the rate of health care cost inflation should be? How should we aim to decrease the inflationary impact of technological practices, and how practically might we get there? The last question will be the main theme of the next chapter, but a necessary first step is to offer some answers to the first two questions. To telegraph my answer to the third question: most of the means to control costs presently used or proposed will work poorly if at all, and in most cases the possible savings are speculative only.

HOW MUCH SHOULD BE SPENT ON HEALTH CARE?

Although it is hard to find any specific efforts among policy experts to answer this question, there seems to be a remarkably consistent informal answer, usually as a kind of throw-away line: "Who knows and who can say?" That may be a wise answer if a specific number is all that would count as a good one, but the same would apply if such a number was sought in any policy area, for instance, education, defense, and environment. But no hard number could be devised for any of them. Yet there *is* a way of achieving an approximation in health care, by asking what signs there are that *too much* money may be currently being spent.[1] Here are three reasons to think too much money is being spent:

- When the cost of achieving health outcomes on a par with that of other developed countries is far higher per capita and as a share of GDP than is theirs.
- When the combination of costs and annual cost growth is doing clear harm to the provision of health care, as indicated by a steady rise in the number of the uninsured, increased co-payments and deductibles, decreasing employer provided health care insurance, and by a decline in the benefits offered by those that still do it; and, in the case of Medicare beneficiaries, rising and economically threatening out-of-pocket costs.
- When there are no sensible, special reasons why the cost of American health care should be significantly more per capita than that of other developed countries.

By those test signs, the United States spends too much on health care.[2] If to those signs is added the fact that the proportion of the GDP spent on health care (16%) in recent decades has far outpaced what is spent on education (6%) and defense (5%)—and a few decades ago they were more or less the same—then one has to wonder if something has gone wrong, and badly so. As a general proposition, I suggest the following: the right amount to spend on health care is what, on average, other developed countries spend (8–10% of GDP), and particularly if there are no obvious special health problems that would suggest that we should spend much more than they do. It is possible to say that the United States has more poverty than other developed countries—an important socioeconomic correlate of poor health—and that is true; and that assessment would justify higher spending, but not spending of considerably greater magnitude. Of course we have more poverty because we have poorer welfare programs and take care of our poor inadequately. Although it is well known that health care spending is in part a function of affluence, it does not automatically follow that the richer a country is, the better its health outcomes.

Rate of Annual Health Care Cost Inflation

What is a reasonably acceptable figure in determining what the rate of health care annual cost inflation should be? Following the same line of reasoning used above, somewhere in the European range of 3–4% of cost increase per annum as a percentage share of GDP would make sense for the United States, as compared with the current 7%.[3] Yet even the 3–4% range is higher than the growth rate of the GDP in most European countries, which has now hovered in the 2–2.5% range; and that gap is a source of some anxiety for them. The most appropriate goal for the United States might then be a rise to about the same as the GDP growth rate, about 3% a year; that would reflect a financial steady-state health care system. That goal has been advanced by, among others, the CBO and the National Coalition on Health Care.[4] Yet given the likely increase in health care costs when the baby boomer retirement surge is at full force, a 3% to 4% range increase might be tolerable, although just barely.

Target Figure

What should be the target figure in aiming to decrease the inflationary impact of technology? As noted earlier, new technologies or the intensified use of older ones account for about 50% of annual health care cost increases.[5] The other ingredients of inflation are change in demographics, general economic inflation, medical price inflation, and patterns of utilization. But technology is by far the most important, its pattern of utilization the most striking. For the purpose of my analysis, I will work with a stipulated figure of a technology inflation that accounts for 50% of annual cost inflation. What should we think as we look at that number and speculate how to reduce it?

We might begin by looking at the projected increase of Medicare costs as $459 billion between 2007 and 2030. Using a 50% technology figure, approximately $228 billion of the increase can be projected to come from that source. To bring the technology share of the general cost increase rate down from its portion of the projected 7% annual cost inflation rate, from 7% to, say, 3.5%, would require a reduction of $114 billion in Medicare technology costs between 2006 and 2030. Comparable cost figures for the health care system as a whole, projected to rise from the $2.1 trillion 2006 level to $4 trillion in 2015, would require a decrease in the technology portion of $630 billion over a 9-year period, and $1.6 trillion for the overall costs. That is what it would take to have an economically sustainable system, which will have to see a steady-state annual budget or something close to it.

If the country were willing to set as a target baseline for cost management the figures and percentages I have laid out, then the magnitude of the task would surely be staggering but necessary. Yet there is no aggressive attempt to move in that direction, even though the consequences of our snail's pace are disturbing to contemplate. The response to George W. Bush's proposals in early 2007 for Medicare reform suggests the obstacles to this daunting task. On one hand, in his 2009 budget proposal, the president outlined a range of cuts that would save Medicare about $89 billion over 5 years, an average of $17.8 billion a year. On the other hand, his proposal was a total nonstarter with a Democratic Congress. In addition, there are obvious pitfalls in even these calculations. Bush claimed that his cuts would lower the annual budget growth from 6.5% to 5.6%, a 0.9% decrease. However, that pace of decline would have to continue on an annual basis for many more years beyond the next 5 years to decrease Medicare costs to the 3–4% level by 2030. A one-time decrease will be of no real help. Moreover the type of budget cuts the president proposed focused heavily on hospitals, graduate medical education, hospices, ambulance services, physician payments, and home health agencies. It is almost impossible to imagine how a steady dose of cuts of that kind over the years could be sustained without destroying the medical infrastructure. The cost of technology in his scheme, however, was barely touched on at all. Would it simply be allowed to run free? No answer to that question could be found.

President Bush's budget proposal drew an immediate hostile response from Democrats and from a wide range of professional groups and associations, and particularly, hospitals. And there is little doubt that, if the cuts were accepted, Medicare would have suffered some grievous blows. It also assumed the introduction of many forms of privatization, such as HRAs and HSAs, expansion of Medicare Advantage, and increased private sector competition. Yet with a Democratic majority in Congress, the chances of his budget going through in its original form were slim, and adding many market initiatives to drive further privatization did not help his cause.

Yet for all of its problems, the Bush proposal took the cost problem seriously, as the Medicare rules require (even if the long-term Republican agenda was privatization of Medicare). The response to it reveals the central dilemma: how to radically cut the dangerously high spending growth of Medicare while at the same time not gut important parts of the program or move it in an excessively market-driven direction. Put another way, if liberals do not like the harsh cuts and program changes proposed by conservatives and view these as ideologically and medically unacceptable, what kinds of harsh changes would they be willing to tolerate that would do the needed job? Few have appeared, nor do any of the other proposals for health care reform deal directly with that dilemma (see chapter 3).

CAN WE GET THERE FROM HERE? NOT BY AVERTING OUR EYES

One does not have to read the literature on medical technology for long before encountering considerable ambivalence about taking the problem seriously, or evading it altogether, or simply denying it is a serious problem. Because of the innumerable benefits of technology, and of the deeply ingrained belief that progress is an inherent good, not to be stopped, there are many incentives to avert our eyes and hope for the best. Western culture, particularly in the United States, has embraced medical technology in a way that leads us steadily down an economic garden path.

As the French historian Henri Pequinot noted over 50 years ago: "The level of health expenditures is basically a function of the 'medicalization' of the country, that is, the current level of medical technology and the psychological expectation that a population has with respect to the consumption of medical services."[6] Another French historian, Patrice Bourdelais, who cited Pequinot, adds that "the higher the standard of living and the better the sanitary conditions, the higher the consumption of health care—and the tendency is always to grow."[7]

Those two historically pertinent observations help to make sense of the ironic fact that the healthier we become as a nation, the more we spend on health care; and there is no evidence at all that, unless forced to do so, we will readily accept spending less, or even just standing still. Yet another historian, this time American, adds a nice touch here.

> By the late twentieth century, Americans knew what progress was: it was more, and then more still—more people, more things, more comforts. By pointing out that more also meant more pollution, more cancer, more extinctions, and more crowding, critics scored points. But they did not reconcile people with a future that redefined progress as a search for less. *Small Is Beautiful* had its day, but it was a short one. Americans seemingly still wanted more; they now, however, recognized that they might not be able to afford it. This was not a change of values. Most people did not feel liberated; they felt deprived."[8]

Yes, Technology Costs Are a Problem, But . . .

As noted above, the obstacles to taking technology costs seriously are formidable. Many physicians seem simply to reject cost as a consideration, and most, in my experience, are at least ambivalent. The historically deep tradition of individual patient welfare does not fit well with the control of costs.[9] The rejection of cost considerations can happen at two levels, that of the introduction of new and expensive technologies into the health care system, and at the bedside with individual patients, with both old and new technologies. Commenting on an expensive new drug, Clopidogrel—used together with aspirin as an antiplatet therapy to reduce cardiovascular morbidity—Dr. Alastair J. Wood of Vanderbilt University, classically using the traditional language of patient welfare, rejected altogether the notion that cost should be a consideration: "to abandon the search for new therapies by describing them as unattractive on the basis of cost would represent an enormous disservice to our patients and would distinguish attempts to improve patient care from the quest for better automobiles, audio systems, or computers."[10] He did not say how the costs should be paid for.

A study of physician attitudes toward cost effectiveness analysis in patient care found that large majority believed that "there is a legitimate need for cost containment in today's health care environment," and that physicians should play a role in controlling costs.[11] But there was considerably more ambivalence when it came to individual patient treatment. A majority felt that no one other than doctor and patient should decide if a treatment is "worth the cost," and a plurality felt that physicians should offer a medical intervention however small the chance of benefit, without regard to cost.[12]

A telling skittishness can be detected even in those who recognize the cost problem and are willing to identify technology as a main culprit. The distinguished economist Henry Aaron and a colleague make a strong case for rationing technology but then draw back at the last moment: "A slowdown in the advance of medical technology and the attendant flow of therapeutic and diagnostic procedures would also slow the growth of health care. . . . [but that] would be a misfortune because it would mean that humans were deprived of the life-extending, pain reducing, and future enhancing contributions that have defined medical advance."[13]

That kind of argument is precisely why we have the technology cost problem: we cannot bear the thought of having less technology than is now available or of not going on to have more of it. Aaron and Schwatz seem to assume that we can have both endless progress and yet somehow control its costs. But if that progress steadily drives up costs to intolerable levels, is this a tenable combination? Their implicit answer to that question does not inspire confidence. They come out in favor of a focus on marginal benefits, which is sensible enough but inherently vague: "limits, whatever their particular form, will require that some sick people be denied some care that is somewhat beneficial but worth less than it costs."[14]

Let us assume that we can work out the calculus for such judgments: "some care," and "somewhat beneficial," and "worth less than it costs," all present a sink hole of murky concepts. What reason is there to believe that such rationing of the lowest-hanging fruit will make much difference in a budget of hundreds of billions? And what of highly beneficial treatments that may be worth the cost, but simply cost too much, threatening any kind of reasonable budgeting? I know that a Rolls Royce is worth the price, a good value for money, but that does not make it affordable to me.

Another skittish response to the technology cost problem, in effect conceding it and then punting, comes from two prominent health care analysts Alan Garber and Dana Goldman: "policies to reduce the price of innovations have the potential to discourage the introduction of the innovations at all."[15] But that would seem to depend upon how low the prices were, how willing the innovators and their sponsors would be to live with small profit margins and, most important, the extent to which we as a people assume innovation to be a central and untouchable value. If we continue to assume it to be untouchable, then there is no possible way to control technology costs. No less untenable is the notion that, if a technology is worth the cost, it thereby becomes affordable (or alternatively, that we should be willing to pay those costs regardless of economic or other impacts).

Constant growth has long been thought necessary for American business; it is the litmus test for how well a company is doing. Yet if that value is considered a feature of market thinking, it is a virus that infects mainline medical thought in its embrace of innovation as well. Nothing is allowed to stand still in health care; it is always supposed to get better. If one adopts that line of reasoning, the costs, whatever they might be, must simply be swallowed. In addition, if a threat to innovation is considered intolerable, the "more and still more" cited above, some go further and argue that we should not worry about costs all that much anyway. Echoing a stance that can be heard now and then, two economists have contended that it would not matter if health spending reached 30% of GDP in the future. That would simply show that "as Americans get richer, they prefer health spending—longer and better lives—to a third car [or] yet another car."[16]

That fine, but as noted above, the rising proportion of GDP devoted to health care already has much harmful fallout. It *does* matter how much is spent on health care. Yet another economist, Tyler Cowen, conceding the serious problems with American health care, praises the United States as the world leader in technological innovation. We "are driving innovation for the entire world," he contends, and that role more than compensates for our other failures.[17] That judgment works as long as you are well insured and can afford the additional out-of-pocket expenses of health care, which fewer and fewer people can.

FEW STICKS, MANY CARROTS

Quite apart from the various kinds and intensity of efforts to ignore, minimize, or defend the cost of technology, there are many carrots and few sticks to deal with those costs. What could be the largest stick of all has, for 35 years, been denied to Medicare. The program is allowed to cover those technologies and treatments that are "reasonable and necessary," a standard that deliberately denies Medicare the possibility of taking cost into account. Because Medicare reimbursement policy affects coverage in the private sector, it makes a decisive difference for everything else in American health care. Worse still, as two analysts have pointed out, the reimbursement policies have the "perhaps unintended effect of encouraging the purchase of costly technologies that will shape the course of hospitals' program and costs for years to come."[18] On top of all that, the program has for years been criticized for its ready support of technological interventions, especially those that are exceedingly expensive, but not for time spent with patients or other low-tech and low-cost forms of caring.

The denial of cost considerations goes back to the beginning of the Medicare program, and the most common explanation is that pressure from the medical device industry kept them out of the enabling legislation since its inception.[19] In 1989, The Health Care Financing Administration (HCFA), the predecessor of CMS proposed that cost-effectiveness techniques be allowed, that is, coverage be permitted for a technology that is as effective as an alternative but less expensive. That standard would, at best, be only a mild form of cost control. It would not deal with the most difficult problem, that of highly expensive technologies that are considered "reasonable and necessary," where cost alone might be a good reason to deny coverage. In any case, the proposed change was not accepted then nor has it been accepted since—although the CMS sometimes manages to take cost into account indirectly by use of the "reasonable and necessary" standard.[20] In an analogous instance of a congressional refusal to deal directly with costs, the Food and Drug Administration (FDA) allows, in clinical trials for new drugs, efficacy comparisons only against placebos, not against comparable existing drugs. In short, if one wants to know whether a new drug offers some benefits over an old one, no research is carried out to make such a comparison.

Muriel Gillick has made a strong case for allowing Medicare to control the price of "specialty pharmaceuticals," those whose cost is at least a $1000 a month, often more than 100 times as costly as the average drug, and whose growth in expenditures has been 34% a year. Price controls on that class of drugs would be particularly important in holding down the cost of the Medicare Part D pharmaceutical coverage. But the Medicare Modernization Act, which created Part D, does not allow for such controls.[21] Although in principle private insurers can refuse to cover very expensive technologies and procedures, they rarely do so, and when they do, they manage to find a medical rather than a cost reason to justify their denial.

Although there are, in theory, a number of "sticks" that could be used to manage and control costs in many cases, there are far fewer when it comes to two of the most frequently mentioned cost inflators: waste or inefficiency, and geographical variation.

Or perhaps it is more accurate to say that the proposals to do something about these lack bite and specificity because of the complexity of doing so, much as there are no sticks designed to deal with a swarm of bees. It is our culture, moreover, that has much to do with these cost inflators: people in affluent societies are often willing and able to put up with waste and inefficiency, either by defining them as not wasteful at all or by having enough money to ignore them. If one is interested in an accurate watch, an inexpensive Timex can do as well (give or take a few milliseconds) as a Rolex, but the latter sell well to up-scale buyers; and they do not, as far as I can see, consider the higher cost wasteful. Like too much of American health care, with other ends in sight than health, a Rolex is meant to do more than keep time.

MANY CARROTS, FEW STICKS

Of "carrots," to spur the use of technology there is no end. I will simply list some:

- American love of technology, from Jefferson, Benjamin Rush, and Benjamin Franklin through Thomas Edison to Jonas Salk to Steven Jobs and Denton Cooley.
- Technology works: it saves lives and relieves suffering, and innovation develops new treatments to replace earlier ones, and also can make possible the treatment of previously untreatable conditions.
- A widespread conviction that life is priceless, and that it is wrong to decide what treatments are cost-worthy, particularly those that can save lives.
- A presumptive research imperative to save lives, taken to be an obligation, especially with diseases that kill large numbers and have a symbolic status as well (cancer, heart disease, dementia).
- Consumer demand and expectations: more and more, better and better.
- Aggressive promotion and marketing of medical technologies to hospitals and physicians.
- Direct to consumer advertising.
- Influence of medical education and medical culture, science and technology based.
- Increased movement of young physicians into technology-oriented medical specialties: more money, more prestige, easier to pay off student loans
- Ready availability of capital for financing technology R & D.
- Competition in the hospital market place—the "medical arms race"—for the best and latest technologies.
- Prestige and visibility of medical technologies.
- Fee-for-service medicine, rewarding the use of technology.
- Physician resistance to cost-effectiveness considerations with individual patients.
- Better fees and reimbursements for technology use than for talking to patients or sitting by the bedside of the dying.

- New technologies assumed to be better than old; that is what "new" is all about.
- Media enthusiasm for new technologies and for scientific "breakthroughs."
- Drug and medical device industries as good stock market investments and good for the economy.
- "Defensive medicine" as a prophylactic against malpractice charges to show conscientious medical practice: "do not stint on technology," which leaves a virtuous paper trail.
- Health care as a growth industry, a source of new jobs and construction, in great part because of a steady stream of new technologies to be bought, disseminated, and housed, all stimulated by increased patient demand.
- Ideological convergence: as children of the Enlightenment, liberals believe in endless scientific progress, and conservatives prize choice and a profitable technology market. Neither side wants to stand in the way of progress, whatever its downside.
- An unspeakable thought: "the idea that the United States or any other nation should try to prevent costs from rising or to slow the growth of health care spending by curtailing biomedical research or by raising regulatory barriers to the introduction of the fruits of such research beyond what is required for safety and efficacy is sheer madness."[22]

Few other countries could come up with a list of incentives to develop and use medical technologies as robust as those in the United States. Our technology situation may be likened to a plant or tree that has many underground roots, going in all directions up and down and seemingly endless, the worst kind (as any gardener knows) to dig up.

An international public opinion survey of American interest in medical technologies told of the many ways we differ from other countries in our embrace of technology.[23] *We* want more, and *they* are willing to live with less. Compared with European countries and Canada, 66% of Americans were "very interested" in new medical discoveries compared with a European average of 44%. Some 34% of Americans believe that medicine can cure any illness if they have access to the most advanced technology and treatment; only 27% of Canadians and 11% of Germans hold such a preposterous view. Concerning the idea that it would be possible for any government or private health insurance to pay for all new medical treatments and technologies, 47% of Americans held that view compared with a European average of 36%.[24]

Two conclusions by the authors of the study have a special pertinence for this book. American seniors, it found, are more interested in medical discoveries than those from other developed countries. "This combination of high interest and high political participation is likely to make it difficult for policymakers to restrain future Medicare expenditures for these technologies."[25] Their other conclusion is even more unsettling: "either there will have to be a change in the public's expectations about medical technologies, or the nation's leaders will have to take a stronger stand against the public's preferences."[26] That article was published in 1991, but there is no evidence that attitudes have changed at all since then.

A number of recent social science studies have focused on the rise in the number of medical interventions that aim to prolong life. One important study, using cardiac care as its main focus, examined the way in which the diminished risk of medical interventions in the elderly has provided increased incentives for medical interventions of a kind that would have been unimaginable even a few decades ago. One result of what the authors call the "biomedicalized conception of aging" is that perceptions of aging are marked by "expectations of continued health and the successful management of risk in 'normal' senescence."[27] Of particular note is the way this mode of thinking about age serves as a direct stimulus to the use of marginally beneficial technologies: "Because the risks associated with cardiac procedures are lower than ever before ... older individuals, their families and physicians feel able to justify their use even when they believe the benefit to be gained is negligible."[28] The net result is that the age of interventions is going up, whether for cardiac care, for cancer treatment, or organ transplantation, or kidney dialysis, not only to save life but also to bring marginal benefits only.

This trend is intensified by blurring the distinction between treatment for heart disease and its prevention: "As the scientific evidence for ... life-prolonging benefit accumulates, and as the criteria for their use are broadened to include *risk* of sudden death rather than a demonstrated history of arrhythmia or heart attack, their potential to extend older lives become increasingly harder to ignore clinically."[29] An increase in cardiac procedures for the elderly in hospitals is a strong reason for an increase in the proportion of elderly in them. By 2002, 38% of inpatients were over 65 compared with 20% in 1970; and that 38% used 45% of the days of care.[30]

A study of the management of health care cost growth in HMOs found that "the process of adopting medical innovation was primarily driven by external factors outside the control of the health plans."[31] Although both physicians and administrators believed that the potential for improved health outcomes was the main stimulus for the adoption of new technologies, it was reinforced by physician competition for patients and the professional prestige conferred by having the latest and best technologies.

Hovering over those motives was a general hesitation "to alienate physicians, consumers, or employers . . . [and that] made it difficult to manage the environment so as to constrain costs."[32] In addition, there is often a lack of good evidence by which to judge new technologies, and, in its absence, the burden of proof rested with those who might oppose it, and that "pressure to reduce costs was diminished if costs were rising in competing plans."[33] In examining Medicare efforts to control costs, often without success, another study noted the importance of information limitations, the cost and difficulty of tracking the appropriateness of services over time, and the lack of incentives to enforce coverage policies.[34] The combination of cultural and professional values and the complexity of managing and monitoring the introduction and use of technology is intimidating.

Can new technologies reduce health care spending? For many years that has been a commonly held view, and it has been a mainstay of advocacy for increased research funding for the National Institutes of Health (NIH). For the most part, however, the history of the relationship between medical research and health care costs can offer little support for that view. On the contrary, research spending and health care costs have risen together over the years, almost in perfect parallel. Research turns up more ways to treat more diseases and opens more new ways to keep alive people who can be treated but not cured.[35] The CBO offers a succinct summary of the evidence in answer to the question of research and its potential for reducing costs: "examples of new treatments for which long-term savings have been clearly demonstrated are few . . .

improvement in medical care that decrease mortality . . . paradoxically increase overall spending on health care because surviving patients live longer and therefore use health services for more years."[36]

TWO CASE STUDIES:
IMAGING DEVICES AND HOSPITALS

When there is so much cultural support for technology and so many incentives to use it and few disincentives against using it, it becomes all the more important to identify the major drivers of increased cost, to separate out the clear signals from the background noise. There are two good places to look for some examples: fast-growing technologies, and hospital and physician spending.

The medical technology industry, endlessly innovating and aggressively selling, is the necessary condition for technology invention; and it is physicians who are the (almost) sufficient reason for the use of the technology. In recent decades there has been progress in just about every category of medical technology, drugs, and devices. Most have been more expensive than older technologies, most have offered at least some (supposed) marginal medical gain over their predecessors (although comparatively few, save for the drugs, have had a full-scale clinical trial for efficacy), and most have been eagerly embraced by doctors and patients. It is hard to say which categories of innovation have had the most impact, but it does seem possible to distinguish between those that have had the widest use and comparatively moderate unit costs (scanning devices and lab tests), and those used by fewer patients but are individually very expensive (devices and procedures for heart disease, cancer treatments). I will focus here on the former, putting aside the no less fertile territory of cancer and heart disease treatments.

IMAGING DEVICES

Diagnostic imaging would be a good example of the moderate cost, wide-use category. CT scans, MRIs, and PET scans are the leaders here and their use has risen rapidly. The title of an article by Dr. Gilbert Welch and his colleagues at the Vermont VA Outcomes Group summarizes well the story they tell, "What's Making Us Sick is an Epidemic of Diagnoses." "As more of us are told we are sick," they write, "fewer of us are told we are well."[37]

At my last full physical, I had no fewer than ten diagnostic scans and tests, six of which were follow-up assessments for some ambiguous findings from the first round. Did my heart murmur, detected by a stethoscope followed by an echocardiogram turn out to mean anything? No. Did my high and rising PSA score, followed by a cautionary biopsy, show any serious problem? No, just an enlarged prostate gland—"but let us check the PSA level again in 3 months." Did some irregular noises in my carotid artery, also detected by stethoscope and followed up with a sonogram, mean anything? No. Did my slightly elevated cholesterol level show a need for medication? Not now, but worth watching, and some later tests would be advisable. Was my slightly elevated blood pressure being medically controlled? Yes, but come back again to check up on that also. And let's review your new and improved asthma inhalers fairly soon as well. I had two CT scans for a persistent cough, which was traced to a sinus infection. We did hit pay dirt with an osteoporosis scan. Yes, I have mild osteoporosis, was put on medications, and instructed to return in a year or so for another scan to see how they are doing. (While writing that sentence, I realized that I have been lax in regularly using the once-weekly prescribed drug, which, I suppose, makes me part of the compliance problem.) Yet it was a CT scan that discovered my sinus problem. Overall, there was roughly a 20% success rate for turning up a real problem and an 80% rate for eliminating a possible problem.

In no case did I ask for any of those scans and tests, and there were at least twice as many as I recall receiving 10 years ago. Except for the cough, I went in feeling well, came to feel anxious for a few months because of all the follow up "just in case" tests, and finally ended feeling well again. I had the physical because I am a modern person tutored to do such a thing, but also, because part of my professional life requires me to read medical literature, I now have my "annual physical" every 2–3 years (even though I get a reminder from my physician every year). The total cost was approximately $5500.

I was not alone. Nearly 25% of physician spending can be traced to imaging ($24 billion) and laboratory and other tests ($11.3 billion), with imaging showing a 1-year increase of 16% between 2005 and 2006 and with laboratory spending up 11%.[38] Total physician spending grew from $87.1 billion to $94 billion for the same 1-year period, an 8.5%

increase. Efforts to control pharmaceutical costs saw a 3% decline. Yet the decline was not quite as good as that figure might indicate. Congress lowered payments for drugs in a substantial way, but even so the volume and intensity continued to grow and products shifted for "less expensive (or more intensive) ones . . . [and] even though Medicare's fees for these products were reduced by over 20% in 2005, drug spending only declined by 3 percent."[39] From 1999 to 2003 there was a 45% rise in imaging services for Medicare beneficiaries versus 20% for all physician services.

Recent efforts by Medicare to control the use of imaging devices have drawn strong industry protests. A CMS effort to control the use of CT angiography in wake of the introduction of 64-slice scanners in 2005 ran into heated criticism from the American College of Cardiology and the American College of Radiology. They were helped along by General Electric, the leading manufacturer of medical imaging equipment. Critics of the control effort argued that holding back on new technologies could "stifle ongoing innovation," an objection that will become familiar, repetitiously so, in the coming pages of this book. The CMS in the end backed down.[40]

Industry invented the scanning devices and laboratory procedures, has aggressively promoted them, and works constantly to develop improved versions. Physicians in turn have economic and other incentives to use them, and patients (like me) are likely to go along with their physician recommendations, even though our skepticism has been heightened by literature and Internet searches. "Better to be safe than sorry" is the attitude of the day. And, as my physician tells me, it is better to have good information than poor or none to make treatment decisions (he knows I am a philosopher); and information is what scans and tests provide. But that kind of information may come at too high a price, playing to my anxieties.

HOSPITALS, DOCTORS, AND EVERYTHING ELSE

Hospitals could well be called medical technology jamborees, displaying all manner of gadgets, machines, and devices. Some of course are more jam-packed than others, especially the teaching hospitals and high profile clinics and academic medical centers. And they are ever buying the newest and latest technologies, for prestige, to attract patients, and to be economically competitive, providing the latest and the best. In 2006, $648 billion, 31% of $2.1 trillion total health care costs, was spent on hospital care in the United States. About 50% of all capital investments in hospitals are for new technologies, most recently for information technologies. Yet hospitals do not plan well for what they will buy. "CMS and health plan coverage policies largely determine the revenue potential that hospitals can expect to derive from adopting a new technology," two analysts have shown.[41] Sometimes they buy too little technology and sometime too much and "CMS coverage will add to the cost of hospital care but not provide substantial new benefit. . . . both health plans and hospitals find it difficult to constrain physician demand."[42]

Physician preference, combined with local competition among hospitals and a lack of information about candidate technologies among hospital administrators, makes the greatest difference. Few of them make use of firms specializing in technology assessment. Their stance is mainly reactive, waiting for physician requests or watching what other hospitals do. "Organizations that have pioneered technology assessment demonstrate expertise," Coye and Kell write, "but have often appeared hostile to technology because of the need to counter the overwhelming incentives that encourage clinically unnecessary utilization."[43]

Although many previous hospital services, including imaging devices, have moved out of hospitals to ambulatory settings, hospitals remain heavy purchasers of new technology and much more is on the way. Jeff Goldsmith has identified a number of likely future developments that have "the greatest potential for reducing hospitalizations or because they create new service opportunities for hospitals."[44] They include genetic profiling for targeting drugs; genetic diagnosis, testing, and therapy; culturing and grafting of human cells; stem-cell research benefits; remote patient monitoring, including sensory monitoring, wireless broadband, and clinical information systems.

Let me add three final additions to the list of ways in which technology has, save for costs, just about everything possible going for it—and particularly how it feeds on itself. A 2003 study found, unsurprisingly, that the availability of new technologies correlates with large increases in health care utilization and spending. In the case of diagnostic imaging devices, the availability of new technologies did not necessarily lead to a decline in the use of older ones; in fact, just the opposite. Most interesting perhaps was the finding that, while large increases in availability led to larger overall spending, that factor could not be traced to any one given technology; all appeared to increase, as if they fed on and nourished each other.[45]

Another study found that costly new technologies stimulate increased insurance coverage, while improved coverage stimulates increased costs.[46] A Pennsylvania study found an oversupply of five medical technologies in that state: lithotripsy, MRI, cardiac catheterization, organ transplantation, and neonatal intensive care. But the study discerned that it was hospital competition and physician pressures that were heavily to blame. Efforts to deal with the situation by a mixture of regulatory controls and competitive market incentives failed, resulting in "excess capacities in all five services."[47] Which technologies will raise costs and which will lower them is unclear. What is certain, however, is that most will be introduced without prior economic analysis.

The costs of technology can in principle be controlled in a variety of ways and at different points in the life cycle of technologies. One set of possibilities is in the evaluation and acceptance of new technologies. Muriel Gillick, making good use of the example of the left ventricular assist device (LVAD), an expensive technology for managing heart failure, notes three intervention points for new technologies: at their initiation, as they are being developed; when they are actually adopted for use; and when efforts are made to disseminate them.[48] In the instance of the LVAD, much of the basic research was supported by the NIH, adopted by device manufacturers, and then vigorously marketed by them. At each stage, there was political and corporate pressure to develop the device in the face of some skepticism based on cost considerations, and a concerted selling campaign once adopted. As it turned out, the high cost of the device led to a smaller market than anticipated, but that was a surprise to all.

Aaron and Schwartz have offered some criteria for another category of technology evaluation, that of improved technologies, not new ones. Using imaging devices as their example, they offer six ways of doing so. Does it work as intended? Is it clinically accurate? Does it alter the clinician's diagnosis? Does if affect the patient's treatment? Do the changes in the treatment of patients improve their health? What are the social consequences of the test, e.g., is it cost effective in comparison with other procedures?[49] And then of course it is possible to evaluate a technology well after its introduction to assess its long-term consequences, medical and economic. It is now rare for a technology to be reassessed, but "the operative rule should be that once is not enough, and both monitoring and reassessment of technology should be part of an ongoing process."[50] There is more hope than realism in that otherwise sensible judgment.

TACTICAL SCHEMES FOR CONTROLLING COSTS

I want now to turn to a number of specific means to control costs. I call them tactical because they are usually presented as discrete methods to be deployed, usually without a specification of what kind of heath care system they might best be used in. My examination will have two parts. First, I will, in summary form, present my own judgment on some of those proposals that are most advanced these days. Then I will move on to a more detailed analysis of a few of them.

REDUCTION OF WASTE, INEFFICIENCY, AND GEOGRAPHICAL VARIATION

This is a most difficult category to deal with because of its diffuseness (like trying to keep dust out of a drafty house next to a desert) and the lack of any unified levers of control to force change. Estimates of cost savings for all three together range from 30–50%, but of course those are estimates only. I have found no very promising ideas for effectively dealing with them.

MEDICAL INFORMATION TECHNOLOGY

Such technology is one of the most popular current ideas, with some decent estimates of costs to put it in place and varying estimates of potential savings, mostly optimistic. But the cost of doing so will be very high (with uncertainty about where the money will come from), and it will take many years to place in operation. I take up this topic in more detail later in this chapter.

Evidence-Based Medicine and Accompanying Clinical Practice Guidelines

The trend in recent years with EBM has been to shift the emphasis from cost control to improved quality. Because many of the findings of evidence-based medical research have often shown medical underutilization of drugs and diagnostic procedures, if current recommendations for physicians were followed, costs could be increased as well as decreased.

Reduction of Medical Error

It has been estimated that 90,000 lives a year are lost because of medical error, and many thousands of others injured (and with the attendant costs of treating its victims). Because other countries have much lower rates of error, it is surely possible to lower ours, and organized efforts are under way to do so.

Disease Management Programs

Such programs are growing in number and promise to lower costs and improve quality. There is considerable medical agreement that specialized programs have good outcomes, but I have not found very specific estimates of what the cost savings might be.

Better Management of Critically Ill and Chronically Ill Patients

Patients in this category are the most expensive of all, but reducing the costs of their care is a neglected area of research. Much of the present work focuses on better integration of care, which is more a quality than cost issue, even if is recognized that the present fragmentation of care is highly expensive. The possibility of cost control here is uncertain.

Wellness Programs and Accompanying Behavioral Incentives

Many businesses are introducing prevention-oriented wellness programs to help their employees lead healthy lives, and some are making use of financial and other penalties for those who do not take care of themselves. The primary motive is to reduce costs, by lowering employee health care costs and absenteeism. No reliable figures have been generated to estimate what those savings might be.

REDUCTION OF MALPRACTICE INSURANCE AND AWARDS

Although malpractice insurance costs for physicians, and high awards in successful law suits, have been a long-time source of complaint, the most general estimate is that only about 5% of overall health care costs can be traced to that source. Moreover, it has long been said (but backed by no hard data) that defensive physician behavior is much shaped by a fear of law suits and that a solid record of the use of technology (e.g., diagnostic scanning) is a main line of physician defense. No doubt there is some truth to all this, but it is hard to project cost savings if that defensiveness were reduced.

CO-PAYMENTS AND DEDUCTIBLES

I put these in their own category not only because they are old and well-used but because they are on the increase these days, in both the public and private sector. We know they have two effects. One of them is that they do reduce health care demand (which can be good and bad depending upon how heavily it is used), and the other is that they shift costs from the government (as in the case of Medicare) and from employers (by using insurance plans that are lower in cost by virtue of the degree to which they are used). The famous Rand experiment in the 1970s is evidence of the former, and present Medicare policies and standard insurance policies increasingly make use of them. Their real impact will depend on the next category.[51]

PREVENTION

Prevention has been a long-time favorite for cost control. It seems self-evident that, if disease can be prevented in the first place, the need to treat will subsequently be averted. But it is not that simple, and studies of prevention show that in some cases preventive efforts can save money, whereas in other cases, it can cost more money than it is worth. Much depends on the particular prevention and target population.[52] With some conditions, such as prevention of obesity, costs can be reduced at earlier stages in life, but the long-term costs of health care are greatest for the nonsmoking, nonobese.[53]

EVIDENCE-BASED MEDICINE

Beginning nearly 20 years ago, the concept of EBM caught on rapidly, becoming an important movement in health care. Originally its aim was broad, to give physicians good scientific information on their diagnostic procedures and treatments and thus to improve patient care and to help control costs. With that information in hand, clinical guidelines for "best practices" could be developed to guide patient care. Although the cost aim was originally secondary, it was present then but has now all but disappeared. The most common definition now of EBM is that it is the "conscientious, explicit, and judicious use of current best evidence in making decisions about the care of individual patients."[54] Although a leading journal in the field, *ACP Journal Club*, reviews a wide range of medical journals for information on EBM, it only now and then cites studies showing that one treatment is more cost-effective than another. The overwhelming research in the field is diagnostic and treatment efficacy. An Institute of Medicine study, focused on gathering and assessing evidence on clinical effectiveness, includes a consideration of "costs of treatment and the economic burden of disease," in a section on "Setting Priorities." But cost is not a main emphasis in comparison with the improvement of clinical outcomes.[55]

As matters now stand, there are many agencies and groups that are interested in technology cost evaluation, but they are scattered, and there is no single, unified source to get such information. There have been proposals to establish an independent organization to study both efficacy and cost issues, but so far that has not happened.[56] Yet there is one feature of the results of clinically oriented EBM that has important cost implications. Many well-regarded diagnostic and therapeutic procedures that have passed EBM standards are not in fact being used nearly as much as they should be: flu vaccine, thrombolytic therapy, pneumococcal vaccine, cholesterol screening and treatment, diabetes screening, and treatment for hypertension.

To get utilization near the 100% level would of course raise costs in the short run even if they might lower them in the long run. One of the failures of the guidelines developed from EBM is that there is a high rate of nonadherence, the practice a victim, among other things, of debates about its methodology, of physician resistance to imposed treatment rules, and of the gap between statistical results drawn from a wide range of patients and the treatment of individual patients.[57] That leaves me with the unhappy thought that if, some day, there were solid economic data on costs and good guidelines for their use, the practice would run into similar obstacles, and perhaps be all the worse given the resistance among many physicians in even taking cost into account in treatment decisions (although pay-for-performance could make a difference).

INFORMATION TECHNOLOGY

Twenty years ago, EBM was seen as the panacea for better management of costs. Twelve years or so ago, the HMO was heralded as the new panacea. Ten years ago, it was cost-effectiveness theory being touted. Along the way many of the other ideas listed above made their appearance, and all the while, the reduction of waste and inefficiency played as a kind of background Muzak. The most recent entrant to be considered as a great cure-all is information technology (IT), which has received some uncommonly strong, enthusiastic support. Many other countries started down that road long ago and are far ahead of the United States, but there is now a push to catch up.[58]

The biggest boost came from a 2005 Rand Corporation study.[59] Noting the wide range of potential applications of IT—bearing on patient safety (e.g., potential adverse reaction to pharmaceuticals), efficiency (e.g., reduced hospital stays), and health benefits (e.g., scanning of patient records for needed prevention efforts)—advocates urged immediate government action to begin putting these applications in place, a process which could take 15 years. Acknowledging the lack of solid data to project the potential cost savings that could be realized, Rand developed a series of computer simulations to come up with some plausible figures. And they surely look good: if 90% of doctors and hospitals adopted IT and used it well, the savings could come to $77 billion a year. An additional $4 billion could be saved by reducing prescription errors. But the installation cost of a good system would be, according to the Rand study, around $98 billion for hospitals and $17 billion for physicians. Another study projected higher costs, $156 billion for installation over a five-year period and an extra $48 billion for operating costs.[60]

Those are surely impressive figures, both for costs and benefits, developed by a solid research organization (even if one lifts an eyebrow when noting that the Rand study was supported by major technology companies, such as IBM, General Electric, and Microsoft). But the problem with computer simulations is that they are simulations, not quite a portrayal of conditions of the real world. And in this case, there are many reasons to be hesitant about the optimism. The first is that, although there is wide agreement, supported by efforts in other countries, that government must take the lead in putting IT in place, Congressional appropriations have so far been small, far from the necessary billions. And the experience of those other countries shows that the start-up costs usually exceed expectations.[61] The installation costs are, then, intimidating without providing much reason for us to believe they will quickly be forthcoming in an era of budget restraint for fresh health care initiatives.

Even assuming the money could be found, it is possible that IT could increase costs as well as reducing them—or neutralize gains—and it takes little imagination to guess how that could happen.[62] Drug costs could, for instance, be reduced systematically by finding ways to gain greater use of generic drugs, but they could also be raised.

Genetic research and the personalized medicine based on it, which with various screening techniques could find the right treatment for individual patients, would surely raise not lower costs, particularly by making use of (usually) expensive genetic-based drugs. Improved safety for some drugs could well mean a much extended patient population using these pharmaceuticals. In short, it reasonable to assume that IT could have many benefits, but it is by no means evident that, even if initially well funded, all the projected savings would materialize or that IT would not promote the creation of some new ways of spending money as well. Its greatest advantage perhaps is that it entails no pain or controversy (as most other cost-saving proposals do), and is thus politically attractive.

CERTIFICATE OF NEED

While not much has been heard in the past few years of state "certificate of need" (CON) programs, they represent an important way to control costs and could still do so if given a new federal regulatory boost. Their aim, embodied in 1974 federal regulations, was to foster coordinated planning and assessment of new services and construction, particularly new technologies and hospital construction. The 1974 Act required every state to have a plan for obtaining approval from a state agency before initiating building construction or ordering new hi-technology devices. Unfortunately, the CON program has had a rocky and uneven history. Its federal mandate was repealed in 1987 together with supportive federal funding. In the years that followed, 14 states discontinued their programs, while 36 still have them, and some have retained real clout. Although their original intent was objective analysis of community need, politics has never been absent, whether in the form of local pressures to build facilities and introduce new technologies or expressed in debates about whether the government or the market should take the lead in the way decisions are made. A fresh federal mandate, with teeth, could revive a valuable idea.[63]

Managed Care

Little has been heard in recent years about the potential role of managed care in reducing costs. After a few years of holding costs down in the mid-1990s, the failure of managed care to sustain that pace pushed it to the sidelines as a means of cost control. A look back is useful, however. A valuable 1998 study examined the relation of medical technology and cost growth and the impact of managed care on cost growth or the diffusion of medical technology. It found that managed care, as practiced in the 1990s, did sometimes reduce the rate of cost increase but that, in the face of the "cost-increasing nature of new technology changes," it made little difference. In short, it was at best a finger in the leaking dike.[64]

SWEET AND SOUR

I want to conclude this chapter by, first, taking a look at where the power lies to bring about significant cost control; and, second, with two examples of approaches to cost control, one of which I consider too sweet, more sugar then vitamins, and the other a bit sour but illuminating.

On the first point, I noted in the previous chapter the ways the Medicare program can control costs; these include higher taxes, increased payroll deductions, cuts in patient benefits, higher payments for the affluent under part B, and a reduction of physician and hospital reimbursement. And, if it chose to do so, Congress could establish the use of cost–benefit or cost-effectiveness methods to determine its coverage benefits. In sum, Congress could use the power of law and legislation to do the heavy and unpleasant work, and if the public, the medical industry, and physicians do not like that, all they could do would be to work for political change to get the legislation changed.

That path for a government agency is strikingly different from what happens in the private sector. Although there is clearly some overlap between the public and private sectors, most of the proposals listed above require voluntary compliance in the private sector—and the leverage to bring about change is correspondingly limited, and often does not exist at all (e.g., regional cost variations). Physicians, for instance, have been lectured for years not to prescribe antibiotics for head colds, and to screen for high blood pressure and high cholesterol levels. But they are not forced to take that advice, and too many do not. Doctors cannot easily be forced to install a first-rate IT system in their office (although Medicare may try to impose it on them). One important reason why cost control is so difficult is then obvious: the "private" sector is private and can do, or not do, what it wants—and it has no central management mechanism, which is of course why market proponents like it so much. So, a question I will leave hanging for now, to be taken up later, is this: is it even possible to imagine the control of costs as long as government has no full and real clout to bring it about? Put another way, can it be effectively done without a government-regulated health care system? My short answer to that question for now is: "no."

An Example That Is Too Sweet

I turn to what I call a sweet (too sweet) example of a comprehensive approach to cost control in a 2007 report issued by The Commonwealth Fund, a long-standing source of solid analysis of American health care.[65] It offers a cluster of six areas for improvement "for slowing the growth of health care expenditures": "1) increasing the effectiveness of markets with better information and greater competition; 2) reducing high insurance administrative overhead and achieving more competitive prices; 3) providing incentives to promote efficient and effective care; 4) promoting patient-centered primary care; 5) investing in infrastructure such as information technology; and 6) investing strategically to improve access, affordability, and equity."

The report looks for policies that, among other things, "have a likelihood of significant reduction in expenditure levels . . . or achieve a net improvement in value." It goes on to list a number of reasons, correctly enough, as contributors to "high levels of U.S. expenditures, inefficiency, and waste." As for technology, it notes that among the factors that contribute to long-term expenditure increases is "the introduction of new technologies/innovations without comparative information on clinical outcomes or cost-effectiveness to guide decisions on adoption and use." That is all the report says about technology.

I have no complaint about its list of targets, solid and sensible enough, but the proposed solutions are at such a high level of generality that it is impossible to imagine how, taken as a group—and so heavily dependent upon the private sector for implementation—these can be achieved; and the fact that many have been around for decades now to little avail should give us a clue. Waste and inefficiency are obvious targets, but there are no system-wide strategies offered to deal with them. Complaints about "Overuse, inappropriate, or ineffective use of care," are surely correct. But in the hodge-podge of a mixed private and public health care system, there are no common levers to deal with these either. Exhortation directed to everyone in general, but the responsibility of no one in particular, is a known formula for failure. National affluence and heavy spending on health care have long gone together, but waste is a standard feature of such societies; and the United States is a leader in that department as well. Getting rid of waste in health care has decades of ineffective gestures behind it but no serious programs to do so. There is, the report says at the end, "a compelling need for a coherent public and private sector strategy, with all parties working in concert toward agreed-upon health system aims." But how is this to come about, and what will it take to make it work?

A later report, by the Commonwealth Fund Commission on a High Performance Health System, focused in more detail on 15 federal policy options for reducing cost increases.[66] It encompassed all the proposals in the Commonwealth report noted above, and then some, but also worked out projected dollar values for the possible savings. It is a valuable report, but it does not itself try to sketch out a strategic plan for implementing the policy options. Yet by simply listing options, a useful enough exercise, it has done no more than—like a poor recipe for making soup—listed ingredients without mention of how much and added at what point in the cooking. The ingredients themselves surely make the end result sound valuable, but without some attempt to set some priorities among them, to assess their political feasibility, to chart regulatory and legislative paths to achieving them, and to consider possible trade-offs if some seem too utopian, they do not take us far down the necessary road. They tantalize us but lack direction and momentum.

An analogous omnibus set of excellent recommendations for Medicare cost-control by well-established health care analysts, Joseph R. Antos and Alice M. Rivlin, suffers from the same kind of problems, that of too much to be done in too many areas of health care with no priorities or clear ideas about how to achieve them. Most would require Congressional action, a difficult road to go down. Taken as a whole, they are exhausting even to think about, but the collective likelihood that all the reforms could be achieved, or even most of them, is not likely, particularly when most are known and of long-standing, persistently resistant to serious change.[67] If there is no magic bullet for controlling costs, it is not evident that the use of a shotgun would prove any better, particularly when there seems to be only Congress to pull the trigger.

A Sour Example: The Metabolic Syndrome

My sour example—revealing, but tart rather than sweet—is a 2006 study of a rise in Medicare spending on chronic disease. Its aim is to "examine the impact of the rise in treated disease prevalence and spending per treated case on the growth of health care costs incurred by Medicare beneficiaries."[68] It builds on earlier data showing that a decrease in the number of people with disabilities might not curb the persistent growth in spending. An important reason for this judgment is an increase in spending by the nondisabled. The case study offered bears on what is called the "metabolic syndrome," each component of which is amenable to a technology treatment. By that label is meant the presence in a person of at least three of the five following conditions: abnormal glucose levels, low HDL cholesterol, elevated blood pressure, high triglyceride levels, and abnormal obesity. Those with the syndrome have an increased risk of carotid and coronary disease. One finding was a sharp rise in treatment in recent years for two or three of the conditions as well as a rise in those being treated for three of them. Most important, "virtually all of the growth in Medicare spending from 1987 to 2002 can be traced to the 20% increase in the share of Medicare patients receiving treatment for five or more conditions during a year."[69]

The painful and mixed blessing outcome of providing those treatments is that, to the extent that they reduce over cardiovascular mortality, "spending may continue to rise, as increases in longevity for people with chronic conditions prolong the period over which they incur high costs year in and year out. . . . mortality reductions resulting from improvements in chronic care may improve health . . . and increase spending simultaneously."[70] Two commentators on the study add another twist of the knife: "ultimately, it will be difficult to distinguish undertreatment from overtreatment."[71]

In their response to that commentary, the authors note that diagnosis of metabolic syndrome has increased the number of patients eligible for treatment. They conclude by noting the importance of three factors "underappreciated in previous work on rising health care spending: the increase in the incidence of disease . . . rising rates of medical intervention, and changing clinical definitions of disease . . ."[72] To these I would add the obvious: the direct causal agents for cost increase are the technologies brought to bear in response to them. There is little in the Commonweath Fund report or the Antos and Rivlin book that directly addresses problems of this kind, which surely pose some serious puzzles in trying to control Medicare costs, or for that matter all health care costs. Ineluctably we are brought back to the deepest of all dilemmas: what are we to do when those half-way technologies that Lewis Thomas wrote about many years ago offer no cures but allow life to continue, propped up by technology, increasingly expensive, for more and more years?

I have in my research found little to inspire optimism about the management of costs and especially technology costs. It invites ambivalence, evasion, moral uncertainty, and close to policy paralysis. But the problem is in principle solvable. As we will see in the next chapter, other countries have done so even if they are having their own anxieties along the way. But "in principle" can seem meaningless in the face of an armada of values, interest groups, and popular appeal all working in the opposite direction. Sisyphus hardly had it worse.

CHAPTER 3

※

GETTING SERIOUS
ABOUT COSTS AND TECHNOLOGY

To use a boxing analogy, most of the actual and proposed means of controlling costs amount to feinting, dancing, jabbing at the problem, not striking with any force. They sound good, and some would surely be helpful, but most of them tend to be general and vague, and some exhibit a paralyzing fear of bursting the technology innovation bubble: "more, just more." Are they the best we can do—or are willing to do?

That last question brings to mind another old boxing expression used when, somehow, the whole match looks fishy: is it possible that "the fix is in"? Do we have a culture, a medical profession, a medical-industrial complex, and an enthusiastic public, that has placed its bet on technology and wants to make sure it does not lose? The obvious answer would seem to be "yes." But what if it is crucial for the long run that the golden-haired favorite not win, that the despised or dismissed contender—the one who looks a bit grim and hardly as pleasing as the crowned champion—is actually the most deserving?

The aim of this chapter is to see what the serious contenders look like. What might actually work to control costs, and in a decisive and major fashion? Any approach to answering those questions must, I believe, be strategic in its outlook, showing the way an ensemble of tactics could work and affect the way the health care system as a whole is run. No country, or region of a country, has found one decisive tactic that solves the cost and technology problem. The wide range of minimalist tactics examined in the previous chapter do not provide individually, or even collectively, any strong likelihood of success for bringing the rate of annual cost increase down to the level of annual GDP increase. A dozen or more speculative ideas patched together are just a large set of speculative ideas.

What would count as "working?" I propose four broad standards: (1) that a variety of proven tactics to control costs are knit together in a way that has effectively held increases down for an entire country over an extended period of time, measured in years; (2) has done so in a way that has been accepted by the public; (3) and has generally commanded a consensus among different political parties and ideologies. I use those criteria for cost control of entire health care systems. But there is also a slightly different definition of success appropriate for the control of technology-driven costs. It is all of the criteria just cited plus one other: that it has (4) controlled technology costs in ways that have done no significant harm to the health of a national population.

To discover what methods are successful in many places, however, does not show they will work in all places. Local and national culture and politics can make certain methods unacceptable. But if so, then that same culture and politics will have to endure the consequences. The first step is simply to look at what works according to the proposed criteria. The previous chapter surveyed actual or proposed discrete individual policy means of managing costs at what I called the "tactical" level. This chapter will focus on the *strategic* level, by which I mean the place and deployment of those tactics within health care systems.

I conduct my examination in three stages. The first is a sample survey of the place that leading analysts, reform groups, and presidential candidates have given to cost control as part of their health care reform proposals. The second examines at the experience of Western European countries and Canada in the control of costs, and the means by which they manage technology. The third looks at some economic techniques that have been used or proposed to control or ration technology.

HEALTH CARE REFORM PROPOSALS

Any number of health care reforms, incremental and total, have been proposed in recent years. A central feature of almost all of them is to eliminate, or significantly reduce, the number of uninsured. Because steadily rising costs are an important reason for the rising number of uninsured, and because the cost of technology is acknowledged to be the most important ingredient in overall cost increase, one might naturally expect a consideration of two points: the necessity in general of cost controls as a part of any serious reform proposal, and the importance in particular of the control of technology costs. With few exceptions, one's expectations will be disappointed. The whole subject of costs is either evaded altogether or, if taken up at all, is usually handled in ways that are as hopeful as they are vague; numbers and careful projections are somewhere between scarce and nonexistent.

As of this writing, Barack Obama has just been elected president. Nonetheless, I think it useful to take a look at the way the other candidates, as well as others, took on the problem of costs. One or more variants of this spectrum of ideas are almost certain to reemerge in 2009 with a new Congress and a new president. I cannot pretend here to do justice to the full scope of the various proposals, much less to judge their overall value. I will focus *only* on those features of them that touch on costs and particularly technology costs.

"PLAN FOR A HEALTHY AMERICA"[1]

Senator Barack Obama's health care proposal moves toward, but would not quite achieve, universal health care by building on the public/private system that is currently in place. To reduce the number of uninsured, Obama would "establish a new public insurance program, available to Americans who neither qualify for Medicaid or SCHIP nor have access to insurance through their employers, as well as to small businesses that want to offer insurance to their employees." For those who cannot afford health care, federal subsidies would be available to assist in purchasing either the new public plan or private insurance. Obama would also "create a National Insurance Exchange to help Americans and businesses that want to purchase private health insurance directly," and he would require employers to contribute to their employees' health care, whether by providing it directly or by helping to pay for it. Obama's proposal includes a mandate that all children have health care.

Obama has acknowledged the need to control the cost of health care, but his proposed solutions seem inadequate in the face of the problem's magnitude. Many of his methods of cost control, such as offering federal reinsurance to employers to offset the costs of catastrophic illnesses of their employees, aim to control the costs of health care for individual employers and employees but not for the entire health care system itself. The cost control measures that do focus on total health care costs are limited and barely mention controlling the technology costs. One tactic is to "invest 10 billion a year over the next five years to move the U.S. health care system to broad adoption of standards-based electronic health information systems, including electronic health records."

Obama's plan also proposes to cut "needless waste and spiraling costs by increasing competition in the insurance and drug markets." As I argue in chapter 4, there is no evidence from anywhere in the world that competition among health insurers or other providers will lower health care costs in any strong and reliable way; and sometimes it increases them. In the one instance where Obama's plan does address the cost of technology, he does so by calling for the creation of an "independent institute to guide reviews and research on comparative effectiveness, so that Americans and their doctors will have accurate and objective information to make the best decisions for their health and well-being." It is unclear whether this institute would have the power to mandate its findings, and, without that ability, such an institute would lack full power to limit technology costs.

In sum, Obama's ideas on the control of costs are mainly unoriginal and conventional. His one fresh idea is "to prevent [insurance] companies from abusing their monopoly power through unjustified price increase. His plan will force insurers to pay out a reasonable share of their premiums for patient care instead of keeping exorbitant amounts for profits and administration." Just how this direct use of price controls will fare in Congress is surely an open question, and it is hard to imagine easy sailing for it. The plan speaks of lower prescription drug costs (e.g., more generics), but there is no suggestion of price controls on pharmaceutical products.

Health Reform 2009—Max Baucus[2]

Senator Max Baucus, Chairman of the Senate Finance Committee, announcing that he plans to push health reform office soon after the new president and Congress take office early in 2009, released in November 2008 what he calls "a paper," not a legislative proposal, but a "Call to Action." Its general aim would be to ensure that every individual has

COSTS AND TECHNOLOGY 71

access to affordable health and that this would be facilitated by what he calls a "Health Insurance Exchange," creating a national insurance pool. It will build upon the present employer-provided insurance system abetted by a Medicare buy-in for Americans aged 55–64, and an expanded Children's Health Insurance Program (CHIP).

Pertinent to cost control he would immediately "refocus our health care system toward prevention and wellness, rather than on illness and treatment." The plan "would refocus payment incentives toward quality and value" and invest in health information technology and "new comparative effectiveness research." The plan would also address fraud, waste, and abuse in public programs, increased transparency of cost and quality information, and malpractice reforms.

There is nothing of great originality, or much forcefulness, in such cost control proposals. Apart from going after the discrepancy between the costs of the private Medicare Advantage and those of traditional Medicare coverage, there is nothing of substance on managing the private insurers serving employer-based insurance. Their present competition, not successful in controlling cost escalation, would apparently remained untouched (see chapter 4 on competition).

SENATOR TOM DASCHLE

Former Senator Tom Daschle was to have been appointed Secretary of Health and Human Services by President Obama and was to be given the title of director of the White House Office of Health Reform. Tripped up by some tax problems, he withdrew. Yet his 2008 book, *Critical: What Can We Do About the Health Care Crisis?*, provides important clues to some likely features of the president's strategy.[3] His approach has two major prongs. One of them is that the reform would build upon the present system, enlarging its scope and coverage, aiming for universal care. The other would be the creation of a Federal Health Board, loosely based on the Federal Reserve system, with a variety of functions. Its most important one would be to "create a public framework for a largely private health care delivery system. Its main job would be to develop the standards and structure for a health system that ensures accessible, affordable, and high-quality care." The model for the program would be the Federal Employees Health Benefit Program, part of whose enhanced aim would be to improve competition among the participating private insurers.

The Federal Health Care Board would be quasi-governmental, composed of political appointees and confirmed by the Senate. It would have three functions: first, to regulate the system; second, to promote high value medical care by "recommending coverage of those drugs and procedures backed by solid evidence,"; and, third, "to align incentives with high quality care." It would exert influence by ranking services and therapies by their health and cost impacts," by its regulatory power over government programs--but not over the private sector.

But it is that private sector that is the main problem with the control of cost, and to hope to manage it by recommendations and not regulation is a tactic with little in the historical record to support it. The FEHBP provides, I believe, a poor model for depending upon the private sector to manage costs (see chapter 4, p. 134). Those shortcomings could be offset, however, by Senator Daschle's proposal to have a government program, modeled on Medicare, to compete with private insurers.

"The Healthy Americans Act"[4]

Oregon Senator Ron Wyden's bipartisan proposal is for universal care — one paid for by a combination of federal and employer contributions and implemented by competitive insurers—is the most detailed about the cost issue, although the details are mainly speculative. Insurers will be required to offer "standardized Healthy American Private Insurance Plans," which will force them "to hold down costs," as will measures to reduce employers' and insurers' administrative costs. The Healthy American Act "relies on competition to drive down costs and promote quality. . . . Ultimately under the Healthy Americans Act, the average annual rate of growth in health spending will slow by 0.86% between 2007 and 2016; this will result in savings of $1.48 trillion."[5] The dependence on competition is striking (but see chapter 4).

"Building a Better Health Care System: Specifications for Reform"—The National Coalition on Health Care

Although this plan is not a specific reform proposal, it most helpfully lays out objectives, criteria for assessing alternative proposals, and a variety of options for consideration. Although there are passing references to the costs of technology, the main leverage point would be a national board to "reflect and reinforce a public-private partnership for improved quality." One of its tasks would be to coordinate the development of national practice guidelines as well as to fund studies and assessments of "technologies and procedures."[6]

A tantalizing part of its specifications for universal health care is that of a "core set of benefits," also modeled on the FEHBP. The growth of costs for those benefits would be constrained to bring the rate of increase down far enough to approximate the growth of the per capita GDP, and "that would effectively produce a 3.5 to 4 percentage reduction in the rate of growth in private health insurance spending." There is no mention about just how the costs of technology as part of this reduction would be dealt with, although the plan would set limits to increases of insurance premiums, a strong proposal that could force a constraint on the use of technology.

AMERICAN MEDICAL ASSOCIATION

The AMA's plan "retains a market-based approach to health insurance coverage. . . . Only when individuals, rather than employers, have the ability to select and own health insurance, will there be increased stability in the system." It is, in short, a market-oriented, consumer-directed plan, with enhanced competition among insurers, "including price, benefits offered, and their willingness to deny services recommended by physicians." There is no mention of the cost of technologies, or of cost control in general, other than an implicit confidence in market practices to do the tough work.[7]

"HEALTH CARE VOUCHERS—A PROPOSAL FOR UNIVERSAL COVERAGE"

This plan, advanced by Ezekiel Emanuel and Victor Fuchs, would provide every American with a "voucher that would guarantee and pay for basic health services from a qualified insurance company or health plan." It would be paid for by a VAT, leave individuals and families free to choose among competing insurance programs, and allow private purchase of health care outside of the basic package. It would eventually phase out Medicaid and Medicare, as well as leading to a likely fade-out of employer-based coverage. It singles out the technology problem only to the extent of proposing the establishment of an independent "Institute

for Technology and Outcomes Assessment." Its focus would be on assessment, but it is left unclear whether its findings would be made man-
datory. Competition among competing insurers would be the main
means of cost control.[8]

PUBLIC OPINION

An August 2008 survey by the Kaiser Family Foundation, after some
fluctuation in earlier months, found that health care came in fourth
(16%) as the dominant issue for voters, after the economy (49%), Iraq
(25%), and gas prices (18%). Yet the survey also revealed that 24% of
Americans struggle to pay for health care, and that it ranked above paying for food, debt, or paying rent or mortgage. The economic downturn
in the mid-2007–2009 period was especially hard on the sick, the uninsured, and minority groups. Predicting where health care as a perceived
problem will be ranked over the next few years can be no more than a
guess at this point, particularly in light of its recent fluctuations. My own
surmise is that it will require a higher intensity of public interest than
the above figures suggest to provide a strong momentum in Congress
after the 2008 elections, though the fallout from the economic recession
may give it some fresh momentum.[9]

   The New York Times seems to me to have been utterly correct when,
in a 2007 editorial surveying the various reform proposals, it concluded
that all of the presidential candidates were evading the tough issues of
cost control, and the same could be said in 2008 prior to the elections:
"All of the plans, both Republican and Democratic, fail to provide a plausible solution to the problem that has driven health care reform to the
fore as a political issue: the inexorably rising costs that drive up insurance rates and force employers to cut back on coverage."[10]

   In chapters 4 and 8, I flag for greater attention two of the most common features of the reform proposals to control costs, competition, and
technology assessment agencies. There are two additional proposals to
be mentioned, single-payer plans; but they will be discussed later.

WHERE COST CONTROLS (MAINLY) WORK AND WHY

As in the United States, the control of costs has been for many years a
focal point for European reform efforts. The Europeans have for the most

part been successful, and successful over a long period of time. I used the word "mainly" above because of variations in the success among countries and because, although doing much better than the United States, their annual increase in costs, in the 3–4% range per year, is greater than the annual growth of their GDP (but a far more tolerable gap than in the United States). That is a worrisome trend for them.

How do the Europeans (and Canadians) do it? The simple answer is that they do it by government control and regulation. That is done most directly in the tax-based systems (e.g., United Kingdom, Canada, Sweden) more indirectly by government regulation and oversight in the Social Health Insurance (SHI) countries (e.g., Holland, Switzerland, France). Although all these nations ration in some mild ways, the tax-based countries are prone to use waiting lists as a cost control measure with elective procedures, although not for primary or acute care. Waiting lists are uncommon in the SHI countries. The tax-based systems, it seems clear, have greater difficult raising money than do the SHI countries, financed primarily by a combination of mandated employer-employee contributions.[11]

CONTROLLING SUPPLY AND DEMAND

Yet if the simple answer to the question of how the European universal care countries control costs is "government," there is no single method by which that is done. Costs can be controlled on the demand side, aiming to induce patients to spend some of their own money on care, or on the supply side, putting pressure on the providers and purveyors of health care to provide less care. The Europeans have placed most of the emphasis on the supply side, using only cost-sharing on the demand side (but with many exceptions, such as for the poor and elderly), and allowing some to opt out of the government system altogether. Demand-side controls have not proved to be very useful. As two long-time European analysts have noted "cost sharing will reduce consumer initiated utilization, but such reductions will not be effective for cost containment. This is because the main influence on health care costs is service intensity, which is provider driven."[12]

The cost control techniques used on the supply side are many and varied, with different combinations of different intensities in universal care countries.[13] They are much too varied in fact to be laid out here, and I will only list them generically:

- Expenditure ceilings: used for health care systems as a whole, or for regions or provinces ("global budgets," capitation)
- Restrictions on the number of medical students and physicians
- State ownership of medical practice (Germany)
- Negotiation of physician salaries and payments with physician associations
- Reduction in hospital beds and shift to outpatient care
- Control of licensing of expensive technologies, drugs, and devices, and of their diffusion
- Prospective global budgeting for hospitals
- Performance-related payment systems
- Monitoring of physician use of resources
- Budget setting and the formation of mandated benefit packages

As in the United States, control of pharmaceuticals occupies a special place, with considerably more debate, discussion, and varied practice than with medical devices.

On the demand side, cost-sharing is used everywhere, but to greater or lesser extent. It is on the supply side that the greatest variety is seen:

- Fixed budgets for pharmaceutical expenditures
- Price controls, price cuts, and reference prices
- Positive and/or negative lists (what may and may not be prescribed); delisting of covered drugs
- Controlling the number of available products
- Development of a market for generics
- Practice guidelines
- Ceilings on drug promotion expenditures
- Prohibition of direct-to-consumer advertising
- Acceptance of parallel trade: allowing countries to buy drugs from countries with lower prices[14]

The notion of a basic "benefit package" is well established in European health care and is ordinarily created by periodic negotiations among physicians, legislators, and health care administrators and with some public participation. For purposes of my argument, it is notable for the SHI countries that medical necessity, appropriateness, and efficacy are common criteria for determining the benefit package, but not all use cost-effectiveness (much less cost–benefit analysis) as a criterion (although Belgium, Germany, and the Netherlands do). Increasingly, however, cost considerations are important for the acceptance of new technologies, and most European countries have established special agencies or programs to assess technologies and to make recommendations to their governments about them.[15]

It should be obvious from the bullet lists above that just about everything that can cost the government money is regulated in Europe. Although the costs of technologies are understood to be important, even more striking is the way in which everything that leads to cost escalation is watched and controlled. Technology is treated as just one more cost item, but an important one. Control everything else, the reasoning seems to go, and you will control technology as well.

What have been the results? The obvious response is that those countries spend less on health care and, on the whole, achieve better health outcomes than the United States. With some exceptions (e.g., Switzerland), they do so with less technology. There are, for example, fewer MRI and CT scanners per million population in European countries than in the United States (though Switzerland has more of both, and Italy and Germany have more CT scanners). Kidney dialysis is twice as common per 1000 population in the United States. Every European country has far fewer cardiac bypass and angioplasty procedures than does the United States. New drugs, typically more expensive than older ones, are much less prescribed in Europe, and cost-sharing is common everywhere.[16]

An interesting international comparative study of technological change showed the effectiveness of supply-side constraints on the use of technology for heart attack care.[17] Between 1989 and 1998, cardiac catheterization increased to 60% of Americans hospitalized for heart attacks compared with 46% of Australians, 24% of Finns, and 25% to 45% of Canadians. During the same period, the figures for bypass surgery within a year of a heart attack rose from 15% to 19% for American patients, from 4% to 9% for Danes, and remained almost static for Swedes, at around 5% to 7%. Trends for primary angioplasty in heart attack patients increased from 5% to 15% in the United States for the same period versus less than 1% to 3% for Danes and 1% to 3% for Swedes. An important difference between America and the other countries was an earlier start in using such technologies and a rapid advance thereafter. All countries showed, however, a gradual increase in the use of heart technologies, although at a slower pace on the whole than the United States.

Even if growing at a slower rate, European health care costs are on the rise, displaying a steady increase in the use of devices and pharmaceuticals. Even with many controls in place, there is an inexorable upward pressure on health care budgets, although how much of this is attributable to medical technology is not clear. That pressure was sufficient for the OECD to say, in 2006, that "if current trends continue, governments will need to raise taxes, cut spending . . . or make people pay more out of their own pockets to maintain their existing healthcare systems."[18] Those words might have been lifted, almost verbatim, from American projections on the future of Medicare.

That much said, European countries have historically held down cost inflation far better than the United States, and their management of technology is certainly a part of it. Whether the Europeans can continue to do so is something worth watching, particularly because they have been using the toughest policy tools available. Moreover, although American health care prices are by far the highest in the developed world, they do not necessarily represent good value for the money. One provocative study found that Americans paid 40% more per capita for health care than Germans but received 15% "fewer real health care resources," while, in comparison with the United Kingdom, 75% more was spent per capita, but with only 30% more health contribution.[19] But although that data may be new, the reality they report is an old story: the United States has long spent the most per capita for health care, but for just as long, it has trailed many other countries in the health status of its citizens. We are paying more for health care than others and getting less for it.[20]

TWO AMERICAN SINGLE-PAYER PLANS

There have been only two American health care reform proposals that embody many of the tough means by which the European universal care countries have controlled their overall and specifically technological costs; and they have clearly borrowed ideas from the Europeans. One of them is "The United States National Insurance Act (Medicare for All)" [HR 676], introduced by Representative John Conyers.[21] This bill is truly a "single-payer" plan, "with the government, instead of multiple insurance companies and you, paying the health care bills." It would extend the Medicare program to the whole population but would use much tougher tactics than the present program to manage costs. It would cover "all medically necessary services," including prescription drugs, long-term care, and dentistry, among other sweeping features. It would also provide for:

- Specifying annual reimbursement rates for physicians.
- Setting global budgets for health care insurers (annual lump sums).
- Negotiating prescription drug prices.
- Setting an annual lump sum payment for each existing Medicare regional program.
- Setting a capital expenditure budget (e.g., for major equipment purchases).
- Providing a health professional education budget, including physician training programs.
- Permitting patients to choose their own physicians, and without co-payments and deductibles, but with no provision to go outside of the national system for private care (following the Canadian policy, but not that of other universal health care countries, which allow regulated parallel private care).

There are few items in this bill that explicitly deal with technology costs (save for pharmaceutical prices), but by virtue of its other features (e.g., global budgeting), it would force attention on technology as has been done in Europe and force steps to control and limit it.

The other plan is similar. It is the "Proposal of the Physicians' Working Group for Single-Payer National Health Insurance."[22] The authors of this proposal call it a National Health Insurance program, and it would be a "single public plan [that] would cover every American for al medically necessary services." The range of coverage would be the same as in the Conyers bill, and it also would exclude parallel private coverage as well as eliminating co-payments and deductibles. Hospitals would be given a monthly sum to cover all operating expenses, and regional health planning boards would allocate funds for the construction of health care facilities and the purchase of expensive equipment. A national formulary for drug coverage would be created, and pharmaceutical and equipment prices would be negotiated "with manufacturers based on their cost, excluding marketing or lobbying."[23] As with the Conyers plan, there is little or no role given to the private sector or to market mechanisms; vouchers, tax credits, and employer mandates are specifically rejected.

There are no specific comments on technology with this proposal at all. The assumption is that "National health insurance would contain costs by enforcing overall budgets and eliminating profit incentives and not by detailed administrative oversight of utilization." Like the Conyers bill, it seems to assume that the general structure of the plan would automatically insure the cost control of medical technologies. That could be a dubious assumption given physician practices and training and increased public demand for the latest and best technologies. And it is equally dubious to attribute most high health care costs to private sector profits and administrative costs. The Europeans have cost-control problems also, but not for those reasons.

Reduced to the most basic level, the two American single-payer proposals, although not mentioning technology directly, rely on regulation and control of the whole system to control costs. It is taken to be implicit in such a way of organizing the system that costs can indeed be controlled—and the European success with comparable systems lends credence to that view. Because these plans so heavily emulate European policies, which work well, they could be, if adopted, likely to succeed. However, they more closely emulate the tax-based systems than the SHI systems. The SHI policies would more likely find acceptance in the United States, but neither plan would really have an easy time of it in the U.S. political culture.

THREE BASIC TENSIONS: CULTURE,
VALUE FOR MONEY, AND RATIONING

There are three other matters bearing on reform that need to be examined. One of them involves American culture, politics, and public opinion, which is likely to have the most significant impact on the outcome of the reform efforts. Another is the widely held belief that, even if technology is the main culprit in rising health care costs, it is too valuable to curb in any serious way. Still another is the problem of rationing, which would be necessary and inevitable in any serious effort to control, much less to lower, technology costs.

AMERICAN CULTURE, POLITICS, AND PUBLIC OPINION

By a strong majority, public opinion in the United States has long favored both a universal care system and a continuation of Medicare. Only rarely has that positive support, however, been matched by a willingness to pay significant additional taxes or to tolerate a cut in benefits. But this unfortunate mix of political support and financial hesitation may now be changing, at least a bit. The public support for many years of higher Medicare premiums for the affluent elderly (the only acceptable financial reform) has now become a reality, with a sharp increase in monthly payments for Medicare, part B. An early 2007 public opinion survey found that not only did a majority of Americans want universal care, but they said they would be willing to pay higher taxes, up to $500 a year, to get it. That figure would hardly be sufficient, but at least it suggested a move away from a persistent tension between the desire for universal care and an unwillingness to pay much to get it. A 1990 survey found that only 22% of those surveyed were willing to pay even the relatively meager amount of $200.[24]

Yet if there is strong public backing for universal care, there is a parallel disagreement on the form it should take. Surveys during the era of the Clinton reform effort in the mid-1990s found sharp differences about the preferred type of plan the public would embrace. Two leading surveys found that "Polls that offer only one plan as a possible solution often shows majority support for that proposal. But when other major proposals are offered. . . . public support splinters." [25] Another survey found that the public was divided on employer mandates (28%), single-payer (32%), and tax credit strategies (33%).[26] Jennifer Prah Ruger has effectively argued that the Clinton effort failed for, among other reasons, its inability to achieve agreement at the highest ethical level on the moral foundation of universal care and a failure at the lowest level as well to reach agreement about the best kind of technical plan to achieve it.[27]

Once again, the wide range of current proposals suggests the same kind of disagreement. The most basic difference turns on the relationship between the role of government and that of the private sector. The two single-payer proposals are similar, but those that try to blend the public and the private are generally different, with various mixtures. It has of course been clear for some decades now (with roots even more deeply in the past) that Americans are prone to be suspicious or hostile to government, particularly what conservatives call "big government," and that long-standing political strain does not bode at all well for single-payer proposals.[28]

Yet at the same time some government programs, such as Medicare, are popular despite many problems. That exception is no doubt why the single-payer plans invoke the idea of "Medicare for all"—even if, in their particulars, those plans go well beyond Medicare in coverage and benefits and call for a much stronger governmental role. Although it is beyond the scope of this book to take on the problem of health care reform in its full range, history, conflicting interest groups, and public opinion make single-payer plans unlikely and mixed plans much more likely. Both kinds of plans, however, have to compete with what I would call the historical favorite: incremental change only mixing government and private sector ingredients, and a rejection of wholesale reform, or, business as usual, just done a little more efficiently.

Getting Good Value for the Money

If there is a good reason to believe that only the European supply side controls wielded by government power and regulation can work to control technology costs, some economists have argued that there are forms of economic analysis that can be brought to bear to cut through some of the political arguments. Their contentions move in two directions.

In one camp are some economists who argue that, whatever problems high costs pose, in the end, the benefits of technology are "worth it." The Harvard economist David Cutler is in the former camp. He is fully ready to agree that technology does raise health care costs in troublesome ways but argues that the economic value to the economy of the lives saved well justifies the cost of the technological advances: "Innovation that results in more benefits than costs is socially beneficial whether or not it increases spending."[29] He uses, however, a conventional if technically dubious technique to determine the value of a year of extra life, that of willingness-to-pay theory, which aims to determine what people would hypothetically pay to extend their life. His valuation is that of $100,000 a year for every year of extra life.

Calculations of that kind rest on a chain of shaky assumptions and ignore the variation among people in valuing the kind and quality of their lives.[30] Moreover, if the benefits [of innovation] increase spending in a way that increases the number of uninsured, whose health will be worse, this amounts to saying that it is "worth it" to tolerate the eventual outcome. I doubt he would want to say that, but that is part of the trouble with "worth it" arguments, which can lead us down some dark alleys. Nonetheless, the "worth it" argument has some sophisticated supporters and has been used effectively in Congress in support of biomedical research, which Cutler claims is the most valuable of all forms of research.[31] As noted in the previous chapter, he has more recently said that the gains have considerably diminished in recent years with the elderly, onto the "negative side" of the ledger (see page 81).

An ambitious European study in 2008 echoes David Cutler's argument that improved health care is a good investment and worth its expenses despite the staggering cost problems it creates. The study, carried out as a cooperative effort by the World Health Organization and the European Observatory, contended that "ill health is a substantial burden economically . . . [and] that cost effective and appropriate spending on health systems is a good investment that can benefit health, wealth and well-being in their widest senses."[32] Although conceding that new technologies raise costs, it argues that the "policy focus should be less on the costs of technological costs per se than on ensuring that new technologies are appropriate and cost effective."[33] A British study makes a good case that health care spending does improve health outcomes, and that cost effectiveness information can show which technologies are most beneficial and cost-worthy. But it does not address the problem of cost-worthy technologies that are terribly expensive.[34]

If a threat to technological innovation is the frequently invoked demon to be avoided in controlling technology costs, the contention that "new technologies are appropriate and cost effective" seems to me the ultimate siren song. To be "appropriate and cost effective" in no way entails that a technology will be affordable. A health care system made up of highly expensive treatments which passes that test would offer no promise at all of being an economically sustainable system. Ever more expensive drugs, for example, that save lives and slow the progress of deadly diseases, can wreak economic havoc even for those with good health insurance. Increasing large co-payments for such drugs is a major source of the problem. Treatments costing $100,000 or more a year are gaining in number, and those ranging from $4000 to $25,000 a year are growing as well. Instead of the customary $10, $20, or $30, insurers can and do charge 20% to 40% co-payments, quite enough to spell financial disasters for individuals and families. The fact that these drugs may be cost effective is hardly comforting.[35]

Perhaps most crucial, there are good indications that the increase in health care spending in recent years has not brought commensurate gains in American health. Not only are we spending at a rate twice that of general inflation, but the rate of annual health gains is small. The United Health Foundation found in 2006 that there is an actual inverse relationship between cost and quality. Between 1990 and 2000 there was an annual health improvement of 1.5%, while the improvement between 2000 and the present has been only 0.3%. They attribute the likely causes of this stagnation to a continuing high infant mortality rates and to obesity.[36]

The phrase "value for money," or "care that is worth what it costs," are ubiquitous in the health reform literature. I find them chronically ambiguous and not all that useful. In one sense, given the figures just cited, it could be said that we are not getting a good health outcome for the money we are spending. But what if we were? That fact would not make our 7% cost inflation rate sustainable in the long run—unless of course we decided as a nation that better health, always better, is worth any price as long as it was good "value for money." I would say that "value for money" is meaningful only after we have decided how much we have to spend (or decide to spend) on health care; that is, it is relative to our economic resources. If I only have $20,000 to spend on an automobile, I must decide which car has the most desirable features at *that* price. If I have a million dollars to spend, I might decide that a Rolls Royce was indeed a better buy for over $150,000 than a Porsche. If we know *retrospectively* that our health care policies did not get as good health outcomes as those countries that spent less, then we can only work *prospectively* if we aim to reduce costs to the level of other systems. If we have no baseline of comparison, and no set budget, then the concept becomes meaningless. In both senses, however, "value for money" is relative to context.

Good value for money is not the same thing as affordability. If we do not care what something costs, then it does not matter whether it is worth the cost. But if our budget is constrained, then we must care: for it is the budget that sets the baseline for deciding on value. The self-evident problem in the United States, however, is that we have few set budgets, certainly not in our Medicare program or our health care system as a whole. Hence, we have no good way of determining what is "worth the money." If we gain no additional population benefit from spending more money on technology, then we can say it is a poor value for money. However, if we focus on individual benefit only, knowing that some few patients will benefit from a technology, but do not know which ones these are, then we cannot say it is not worth the money; it will be for the fortunate patient who benefits, even if she is in the minority. It is a marginal health benefit from a population perspective but not from a traditional individual benefit perspective.[37] That is the basic tension in resource allocation, and the most painful one.

ECONOMIC TECHNIQUES AND TECHNOLOGY ASSESSMENTS

The other economic camp works with economic techniques meant to offer a more or less value-free (and politics-free) way of determining the value of various technologies and treatments. The assorted supply side controls that limit technology and its use in Europe provide decent evidence that good population health can be achieved with less technology than the United States deploys; and regional variations in the United States reveal enormous differences in technology use, but all of which produce roughly the same health outcomes. Is there a way to cut through all this confusion? All patients, Aaron and Schwartz argue, should "receive care that is worth what it costs. . . . [and we should] eliminate care that is not worth what it costs."[38] That standard, they say, is not being met, even for the well insured. Why not, then, use the cost-worthy principle as a way of assessing and using technology? If that standard were accepted as a rational way of proceeding, a great deal of squabbling over high technology costs might be bypassed, eliminated by what seem to be commonsensical economic principles.

A way into those questions is afforded by the experience of European countries with technology assessment programs and agencies, amply documented in a report of the European Observatory of Health Systems and Policies.[39] It surveys thirteen European countries and provides detailed case studies of six others that have such agencies. Four questions are central to their work: (1) is the technology effective? (2) for whom does the technology work? (3) what costs are entailed in its use? (4) how does the technology compare with available alternatives?[40] While there are a great variety in the agencies and their activities, they generally fall into two categories: "independent review bodies that produce and disseminate [technology] assessment reports," usually of an advisory nature; and "entities under government mandates . . . with responsibilities for decision-making and priority setting . . . The latter serve an advisory or a regulatory function."[41] Although there is general agreement that the work of such agencies should be transparent and represent the contributions of lay persons as well as experts, that is often not the case, sometimes weakening the accountability of their work. The criteria for assessment include, among others, therapeutic benefit, patient benefit, cost-effectiveness, budget impact, and equity considerations.

Central to the assessment work of those agencies are a variety of economic techniques: cost effectiveness analysis (CEA), aiming to find which treatments will cost less than comparable ones but achieve the same or better health effects; cost–benefit analysis (CBA), which uses willingness-to-pay methods to determine good cost–benefit ratios; and cost-utility analysis (CUA), which principally uses quality-adjusted life years (QALYs) to come up with a number that shows the relationship between length of life and quality of life for a particular treatment.

Despite its problems and assaults over the years, the concept of QALYs merits a strong place in resource allocation decisions and is used by all the European agencies. How might we better deal with tradeoffs between a shorter life with higher quality, or a longer life without it? Its specific aim is to compare the incremental cost of an intervention with the corresponding incremental health improvement. No one has come up with a better technique for doing so. To be sure, QALYs runs afoul, even more than the other techniques, of many technical criticisms (e.g., determining what counts as "quality," and discriminating in controversial ways against the old and the disabled), of the difficulties of moving from theory to practice (given the variety of patient values and their even more varied maladies), of the physician bias toward satisfying patient desires without regard to cost, and of persuading legislators and administrators to take seriously formulaic, impersonal solutions to complicated moral and economic dilemmas, not well attuned to fractious legislators, powerfully conflicting ideologies, and the vagaries of human needs and desires.

Yet the idea of QALYs helps us to deal with an important policy question: can we find a way to appraise a technology or to compare various older technologies for their cost-effectiveness that does not force us to radically individualize our judgments about their use? We know, on one hand, that there are great variations in how long a life people hope for and in the quality of life people want or are willing to put up with. We should also know that to leave all decisions in the hands of individual doctors and patients cannot constitute good public policy in the face of scarce resources: the patient, not the social good, is the only focus. The rankings of technologies that using QALYs makes possible because it provides a single metric value (with a range of $50,000–100,000 as a cutoff for costworthy treatment) are its main strength. "Such rankings," David Meltzer has written, "are useful because they suggest that one should always engage in activities at the top of the [treatment or technology] list before moving down the list."[42]

To say that QALYs offers a way out of the dilemma noted above does not mean it can or should be used exclusively. It does offer a way to find a general direction, a presumption for a decision, but one that can be overcome if there are strong reasons to put it aside.[43] The other reasons will have to be varied, subject to particular circumstances and leave at least some breathing room for individual patient judgments at both the clinical level and policy level.[44] But that flexibility should be severely limited in making judgments about new technologies, where the aim ought to be to limit individual judgments. To allow these latter fully in would subvert sensible policy, which ought to be oriented to the common good and a fair distribution of resources. Along with most European countries, the U.S. Panel on Cost-Effectiveness in Health and Medicine convened by the Public Health Service in the 1990s commended the use of QALYs.[45]

Yet the debate continues, not only about the general cogency of QALYs but also about various details in using it. The limitations of the economic technique have, in addition, attracted those who are drawn to procedural rather than substantive ways of making difficult rationing decisions. Norman Daniels and James E. Sabin have been leaders in devising criteria for the public legitimacy of rationing and allocation decisions: transparency of the decisionmaking process; publicly accessible decisions and the reasons in support of them; norms summed up in the phrase "accountability for reasonableness."[46]

It is hard to object to what is patently a sensible and democratic way of making final decisions, that is, decisions to be taken when the arguments have all been laid out, everything heard and discussed, and no more is to be said. However, in dealing with questions as complex as those of health technology and costs, a hardly less important issue is: what *ought* we to be talking and arguing *about*, what *ought* to be the substantive content of the democratic deliberations? "Transparency" as a standard of judgment does not tell us how to evaluate that which is now open for inspection and interpretation. When fundamental questions of, say, "benefit" to patients arise, then we will, or should, be pressed to ask just what is *really good* for people, or necessary for them.

Those are crucial substantive issues, not fully captured in a procedural model. Questions of that kind make Americans uncomfortable, and that discomfort makes a more formal and detached procedural approach tempting, a kind of end run on matters of troubling depth. For all of their technical policy and ethical problems, the use of both QALYs and cost benefit calculations does not allow us to bypass the most troublesome matters. We often just bog down when we try. But try we must. Accountability for reasonableness is a fine standard, but only if partnered with a probing of issues whose depth and scope are often beyond the reach of democratic legitimacy, which helps us live together but does not tell us how we ought to live—what it is we should want, for ourselves as individuals and for ourselves as part of a community. [47]

EUROPEAN PUBLIC OPINION ON COST CONTROL

Because I have cited the European health care systems for their more or less successful control of costs, it is instructive here to take a quick look at European public opinion about the kinds of policies that hold down those costs far more successfully than American efforts. Now a decade old, a comprehensive review published in 1999 nevertheless provides some insight.[48] Two themes stand out. One of them is that, in the face of rising costs and greater demand, there is the kind of ambivalence about paying for these policies that is present in the United States as well. A strong majority, for instance, wants a full range of medical services and care, and a plurality in most countries wants unlimited funding for it, but with a strong minority agreeing that some limits to care should be set.[49] Yet only a small minority approves of higher taxes to keep up with the cost increases. Higher taxes on tobacco and alcohol are a much more popular option than higher income tax, and the most popular of all is that of "lower national spending on other things." In other words, "pick on the other guy."

The other theme is that there appears to be a greater willingness to tolerate rationing and priority setting in Europe than here (with some significant national variations). In the face of a scarcity of resources, the Germans and the Dutch were more willing in the face of resource scarcity to limit care to essential care only than were the French. The Netherlands and Sweden were more willing to accept priority setting than Germany and France. Politically, those who labeled themselves on the right were more tolerant of rationing and priority-setting than those on the left. Although there was evidence of a growing interest in public participation in fashioning health care priorities, there was also a reported "reticence" as well, but it tended to decrease when the public was given good information, support, and responsibility.

Nonetheless, there was a relatively uniform belief across OECD countries that, however important public participation is, rationing and priority-setting should best be left to physicians.[50] I know of no American public opinion survey that has dealt with the question of who should make rationing decisions. Although there are many books and articles on the subject, at least in academic circles there has long been resistance to individual physicians playing the role of rationer. That position is based primarily on the grounds of great variations in the moral and social values of physicians as well as an anxiety that patients would soon become fearful of doctors who could wield that kind of power.

My own inclination is toward what might be called "structural rationing," that is, rationing that is built into the organization on the supply side of the health care system. That approach would mean limiting the availability of scanning devices, ICU beds, expensive new drugs and procedures, and hospital beds, leaving decisions on the use of the policy-limited technologies up to local institutional committees to set the rules for handling the inevitable shortages. Whether the rationing be that of marginally beneficial technologies or those with real, and life-saving, benefits, the institutional or regional decisions would be made collectively, representing so far as possible a combination of technical judgment and community ethical standards. QALYs and the other available techniques would be used as well to help fashion the standards.

Of course the context for such a resource allocation system would be that of the available funds, wherever these might come from. The stringency of the rationing would be a direct function of those funds. A strong argument for government-run or -regulated health care would be to reduce suspicion that the private sector was allowing profit margins and shareholder claims to influence rationing decisions. Government-imposed budget caps would surely be open to politics and interest group pressures, and potential distortion as a result, but there would likely be more transparency in that kind of system than in the private sector. Yet even as a few analysts take on the problem, the whole topic of rationing in America has had a struggle even getting started. Participants in the Clinton health plan work groups in 1994 were specifically forbidden from using the word "rationing," and it is by no means certain that such a taboo has been vanquished. No current presidential candidate has used that word, or even a euphemism for it.

AMERICAN CULTURE AND MEDICAL TECHNOLOGY

As someone who has spent much time over the past 20 years going back and forth between the United States and Europe, examining and comparing their health care systems, I observed on my latest day there what I had seen on my first day. The politics of health care, its values, and its organization reflect two very different cultures. America's embrace of choice and individualism, strong on market values, and Europe's embrace of solidarity, the regulation of choice, and a wariness about the market stand out as vivid contrasts. The difference is reflected in America's more vigorous use of technology, industry's resistance to even assessing technology much less attempting to control it, and the fear that any control of technology could dampen innovation. The European media, while not neglecting health care, pays far less attention to it than in the United States, is denied direct-to-consumer advertising, and does not flood its news with our peculiar domestic cheek-to-jowl mix of exciting imminent cures and terrifying new threats to health. I left the United States the day after Viagra was introduced to the market, an event reported in page one stories in America but barely mentioned in Europe.

In comparing the European means of controlling costs and those used or proposed in the United States, I cannot help thinking that we have the worst possible situation: what works well in Europe to control costs, a strong role for government, is for the most part politically rejected in the United States; and what *is* politically acceptable in the United States, one form or another of organizational reform voluntarily imposed, does not and cannot effectively hold down cost increases.

Well-entrenched cultural patterns are notoriously difficult to change, and for me at least that point has hit home almost every day since I began working on this book. Technology is as deeply embedded in American health care as it is in the American psyche and society, and our national ideological struggles, too often harsh and unyielding, are now as much a part of our health care as they are of our political life. But perhaps I need to quality that last statement. There are profound ideological differences over the management and control of technology, as with health care more generally, but technology is embraced by both liberals and conservatives, although for different reasons, which gives it a particular tenacity. Liberals have characteristically followed the Enlightenment, pursuing scientific progress of all kinds and in medicine no less than anywhere else; and liberals have resisted rationing health care, seeing the process as a threat to equal access. Conservatives like progress as well, but their emphasis falls more on the economic benefits of medical progress and on the right of and the need for individuals to make their own health care choices, unimpeded by government.

Both sides get nervous about any threat to technological innovation, considered to be a fundamental value, not to be compromised and even, it often seems, when its pursuit directly threatens other goods and values, as is now the case. Control of technology costs, therefore, finds few friends and many opponents, even if those opponents often concede it is a serious problem. The common love of both sides for technology is enough to intimidate any reformer.

CHAPTER 4

COMPETITION

THE FIX THAT WILL FAIL

With the advent in 2009 of a new president and Congress, health care reform will obviously be a leading issue. A number of reform proposals have already been advanced, ranging from single-payer plans to those with a varying mix of government and market strategies. The role of competition in health stands squarely in the middle of the debate, cited in a variety of the proposals. A number of economists, political conservatives, and many from the business community have had a long-standing affection for competition; and it is now a key ingredient of CDHC.

In its production and distribution of many goods, competition—from food to airplanes, computers, and cell phones—has brought constant innovation, lower unit prices, consumer satisfaction, and a steady improvement in our standard of living. If competition can do that for many other goods and services, why could it not do the same for health care? Even the European universal health care systems are expanding the role of the market, and particularly that of competition. With the exception of some single-payer plans, most of the recent American proposals for health care reform give competition a central place in the control of costs.

Yet while the attraction of competition is understandable I will argue that competition is too untested, too speculative in its potential national impact, and too great a gamble to ever be depended upon to reliably control costs—and that it has failed in health care far more than it has succeeded. That it may work locally here and there, as I show, does not prove that it will work on a wider national scale; and it could be positively harmful if loosed wholesale as a key part of health care reform. There are, to be sure, many problems with government-run, -dominated, or -regulated health care systems, in the United States and abroad. But these have on the whole been successful, consistently holding costs down better than the private sector and managing to capture popular support as well. Most important for the current American dilemma, the wide range of government plans and ongoing reforms in Europe and the United States offer a rich variety of ingredients that can be drawn upon to assemble a viable, and uniquely American, domestic health policy that can control costs.

EVALUATING COMPETITION

How should competition be evaluated? What are the pertinent standards for judgment? Should it be by extrapolation from its success in the commercial world to health care, as many market advocates tend to argue? I believe that move to be a mistake; commerce and health care dwell in different realms of policy and welfare. Or should competition be favorably evaluated because it is more compatible with the American way of life than the alternative, government dominance and regulation? Yet with 50% of American health care now already financed by government, and steadily rising, no case can plausibly be made that, somehow, government-sponsored activities and institutions are less consistent with American culture than those in the private sector. Or should competition be welcomed because it is most conducive to meaningful patient choice, giving patients a good menu to choose from and forcing them prudently to choose from it? This possibility is, at best, hypothetical, lacking a track record. Or should evaluation be based only on the available empirical evidence and drawn from competition in health care not from other sectors of the economy? This last possibility seems to me the most plausible, and the one I will pursue.

Kenneth Arrow: Is Health Care Different?

A good starting point is for an evaluation of competition is a by-now classic article by the economist and Nobel Laureate Kenneth Arrow in 1963, "Uncertainty and the Welfare Economics of Medical Care."[1] As the title might suggest, it was a technical article, meant mainly for other economists. But the issue Arrow took on was one that has had recurrent echoes over the past 40 years: whether health care is an appropriate locus for market activities.

Arrow's answer was a carefully crafted, nuanced "no." Health care is different from other areas of economic activity, presenting many aspects that will make a make a good medical market hard to achieve. A workable use of the market, based on the best economic theories, that is, perfect or near-perfect conditions, requires many features that health care does not present. The nature of demand for health care is "irregular and unpredictable"; the patient is forced to trust his physician, lacking his knowledge and experience; the customer "cannot test the product before using it"; "recovery from disease is as unpredictable as is its incidence"; and entry into the field of health care is limited by professional and licensing restrictions (anyone can try to make and sell better automobiles, but not everyone can start practicing medicine).

Arrow's analysis was influential in persuading many economists and others at the time that the matter was settled: the market would not work well in health care, particularly if the paradigm was that of a perfect market. The distinguished economist Burton Weisbrod wrote that "we cannot construct wise public health policy on health care by applying elementary economic analysis. Competition does have a role to play. Yet the markets for health care and chocolate chip cookies *are* different." [2]

Two much later responses stood out for me. One of them was the indignant outcry many years later by a leading health economist, James C. Robinson, against the influence of the Arrow article among his professional colleagues: "The most pernicious doctrine in health services research," he wrote, "the greatest impediment to clear and successful action, is that health care is *different* . . . . To some within the health care community, the uniqueness doctrine is self-evident and needs no justification." [3] But food and shelter, he notes, are even more essential than health care, yet they are produced and distributed without the latter's paraphernalia of licensing, insurance, and thousands of pages of federal regulations. Judging health care "different" also blocks many management techniques that could be used in its organization.

A contrasting argument, contending there is indeed a difference, has been developed by another leading health economist, Thomas Rice of UCLA. "Economic theory," he has written, "does not support the . . . belief that [market] policies will enhance economic efficiency, or the more general one that they will increase social welfare. This is because the theory is based on a large set of assumptions that are not and cannot be met in the health care sector."[4] Among the wrong assumptions is the view that consumer tastes are predetermined; that a person is the best judge of her or his own welfare; that consumers know, with certainty, the results of their consumption decisions; that individuals are rational; and that supply and demand are independently determined.[5]

A further phase of that debate came with an exchange between Rice and Mark Pauly, a market-inclined economist from the Wharton School. Rice wrote that "if one accepts the viewpoint that economic theory does not demonstrate the superiority of market forces in health, the important corollary is that all important questions must be answered empirically . . . Market forces may indeed have a prominent place in health care organization and theory . . . but economic theory does not show them to be necessarily a superior approach."[6]

Pauly responds by arguing that even those who embrace the competition model as the best route for reforming health care "do not base that conviction on the belief that economic theory shows the market to be superior to government regulation . . . theory tells us that, at best, the ideal market can tie an ideal government, not that it can do better."[7] "We should," he contends, be talking about "imperfect markets versus imperfect government."

I took away three useful conclusions from the line of thought running from Arrow to Rice and Pauly. The first is that economic theory will not decisively tell us how to evaluate the role of the market and competition in health care, although it may help. The second is that Pauly is right in proposing that we should cast the debate as one between "imperfect markets versus imperfect government." The third is that Rice is right in saying "that all important questions must be answered empirically." I combine those three ideas into one answer to the question to evaluating competition: it is to require empirical evidence to support its efficacy, but without a demand for decisive evidence, only good approximations.

To those three conclusions I add a fourth consideration: competition cannot be judged in isolation from the health care system of which it is meant to be a part. What kind of work is it meant to do, and will that work fit into the overall goals and values of the system and the society of which it is a part? As Stuart Butler, an innovative economist with The Heritage Foundation, has emphasized, success with the market will be a function of public demand, government regulation, and context.[8] Another important economist, Alain Enthoven, who did the pioneering work on managed competition, has cautioned, "everything that sounds like 'competitions' or 'markets' or 'private sector' will not necessarily improve economic performance."[9]

But what does the available evidence tell us?

Examining the Evidence

I examine four places where some evidence is available: at a series of studies in the 1980s and 1990s of hospital and HMO competition; at FEHBP; at a few miscellaneous examples; and at the historical record of the private sector in controlling costs.

If one looks back over the past 30 years or so, it seems fair to say that careful research on competition has been thin and sporadic. A large number of competition studies took place in the 1980s and 1990s stimulated by a growing interest in market ideas during the Reagan years, by constant cost pressures, by the rapid increase in HMOs, and by the early stirrings of CDHC. But they declined after that. Two areas of competition were intensively studied, hospital and HMO competition. I have broken down the studies into two groups, those where the evidence from the studies was favorable toward competition and those where it was not.

I surely do not want to claim that these studies fully answer the question of whether competition works or not in health care. They are just one of the more fruitful places to find studies, otherwise in short supply. That many of them are no doubt examples of imperfect markets is, by the Mark Pauly criterion noted above, no reason to dismiss them. I note, however, that although some studies have tried to assess quality rather than price competition, there are many difficulties in defining and measuring quality.[10]

HOSPITAL COMPETITION

Hospitals are the major center of high cost medicine and advanced, expensive technology. Their ability to manage, or not manage, costs in a significant way is a major factor in national health care. In large urban areas, there are many hospitals, all of them seeking patients and physician referrals, and often creating special programs to do so. One way or another, these hospitals are often in competition with each other, and that reality is worth looking at (although on the surface usually competing on quality not costs).

Hospital Competition:
Unfavorable to Cost Control or Quality

James C. Robinson has been one of the leading economists to study the impact of the market and competition on health care. Using data from 1982, Robinson and his colleagues measured the impact of California hospital competition on the length of stay after surgery for 10 surgical procedures. While controlling for variables, the study found that hospital competition led to longer patient length of stay, and thus higher costs, with percentage increases ranging from 8.4% to 22.9% over lower-competition markets. Robinson and Luft, this time using earlier data from 1972–1982, also examined the impact of competition on California hospital costs. This study found competition to have a negative cost impact. The average cost per admissions and cost per patient-day for hospitals in higher competition markets were 26% and 15% respectively higher than for those hospitals in lower-competition markets.

Jonathan Gruber, using data from 1984–1988, conducted a study of the impact of competition on the level of care a hospital provided to the uninsured. Gruber hypothesized and found, with statistical significance, that prior to 1983 hospitals had a significant source of income because of the near 100% reimbursement for patient services, which was then used to provide care to the uninsured. However, once hospitals were forced to become cost-conscious in order to gain HMOs' patronage, this source of income greatly diminished, along with the level of care provided to the uninsured by hospitals in more competitive markets.[11] Patrick Rivers and colleagues, in a study using 1991 data, found that greater hospital competition was significantly and positively correlated with increased hospital costs across 29 metropolitan statistical areas.[12]

Another study found that in 1982 costs per admission in hospitals with 11 or more neighboring hospitals in a defined geographical market were 98% higher than for those hospitals with no neighbors. Even after factoring in various controls, the difference in costs was still 20% higher in the more competitive markets. Additionally, wages were higher in highly competitive markets because of the plethora of alternative hospitals for employment.[13]

Hospital Competition:
Favorable to Cost Control or Quality

The leading proponents of the benefits of competition in health care recognized that, prior to 1983, competition did not show the expected cost-reducing effect. In 1983, however, California introduced legislation to support procompetitive practices, and Medicare initiated its prospective payment system (PPS). A difference between the pre- and post-1983 eras was expected and it appeared.

Glenn Melnick and Jack Zwanziger found that from 1983 to 1985 in California there was an increase in inpatient costs of less than 1% for hospitals in low-competition markets, whereas for those hospitals in high-competition markets, inpatient costs decreased by 11.29%. Additionally, after controlling for the effects of Medicare's PPS program, there was a 3.5% reduction in the rate of increase for inpatient cost per discharge. In a broader survey of hospital competition, they found "a dramatic slowing of rates of increase in costs for hospitals in more competitive areas . . . "[14] A 2000 study examined data from the mid-1990s from Washington state to determine the impact of competition on hospital prices. The study's results showed that, in more competitive markets that offered prospective payment plans, a hospital, based on the level of competition, was more likely to assume a greater amount of risk when accepting payment plans.[15]

Along these same lines, Town and Vistnes examined Los Angeles data from 1990 to 1993 and found that a hospital's bargaining power and price decreased as contracting options increased for HMOs in the market region.[16] Gowriskaran and Town also found that, as hospital competition increased for HMO patients, hospital prices decreased and hospital quality (based on risk-adjusted mortality) increased. But the study also found that, for government regulated services such as Medicare, as competition increased, the level of hospital quality decreased. Gowriskaran and Town claim that HMOs cared both about the price and quality of the hospital with which they contracted, and thus that this competition was beneficial to healthcare.[17]

Two other studies located a positive effect of competition on nonprice factors, such as quality, an issue of concern among anticompetition voices: if price begins to decline as the result of competition, will the quality of care go down as well? Rivers and Fottler, using 1991 data, studied the impact of hospital competition on quality of care as indicated by risk-adjusted mortality rates. They found a statistically significant and positive relationship between hospital competition and quality of care; as the level of competition went up, risk-adjusted mortality rates decreased.[18] Rogowski et al., examining data from California, also found that increased hospital competition for HMO contracting had not led to a deterioration in quality of care and that hospitals were not just competing on price.[19] Bemazai et al. found that hospitals in high HMO penetration areas showed a statistically significant lower rate of cost growth from 1989 to 1994.[20] However, these results were only significant in the most competitive of markets.

A comparison of the changing effects of competition on nonprofit and for-profit pricing behavior in California from 1986 to 1994 found that market concentration changed over that period with prices higher for nonprofit hospitals in less competitive areas.[21] The authors of the study also noted that nonprofit hospital mergers led to higher prices, not lower ones, and that the price increases resulting from nonprofit mergers getting larger over time.[22] Thomas Bodenheimer has noted that "competition can reduce health care costs under favorable conditions. Those conditions existed for a brief period in the 1990s."[23] He goes on to note that "the consolidation of health plans and hospitals may have put an end to that brief competitive era.[24] James C. Robinson, who has also followed the history of mergers, points out that an important reason for a decline in competition is "that there have been no major innovations in product design and organizational structure" that could enable newcomers to compete with the advantages of incumbents. And those incumbents are more interested in using their market power to consolidate market power than to stimulate competition.[25]

HOSPITAL COMPETITION: REGULATORY VERSUS COMPETITION STRATEGIES

A few studies have compared regulatory and competition strategies for controlling costs.[26] One study examined data from Minneapolis and Baltimore to compare the impact of competitive and regulatory strategies on health care costs. From 1971 to 1990, the annual rate of hospital cost increase in Minneapolis (procompetition) was 10.0%. Baltimore (proregulation) during that time period had an increase of 10.5%, whereas the national average was 11.2%. In 1990, Baltimore's cost per discharge was 6% lower than the national average, whereas it had been significantly above it in 1976. Overall, these data, without great statistical significance, showed a negligible difference between the differing regulatory and competition strategies.[27]

Robinson and Luft compared average hospital costs per admission from 1982 to 1986 for the market-oriented strategies of California compared with the regulation-oriented strategies of New York, New Jersey, Massachusetts, and Maryland. California's average rate of inflation was 10.1% lower than the national average. Massachusetts and Maryland experienced even lower rates (16.3% and 15.4%, respectively), whereas New York experienced a 6.3% reduced rate of inflation compared to the national average, and New Jersey experienced a rate comparable to the national average. Although the authors do note that California's data are only significant in highly competitive markets, these data reveal that both strategies have similar effects on the healthcare market.[28]

Zwanziger and Melnick, whom we cited earlier for their finding of the value of competition for California hospitals, wisely noted that although both regulation and competition can lower cost increase, "the 'cost' of cost containment is relevant . . . in the long run, cost control that degrades quality or access excessively will become unacceptable, both politically and otherwise."[29] A particularly provocative article by Shortell and Hughes in 1988 provided some evidence that patient welfare was at risk in both highly regulated areas and for those admitted to hospitals in relatively competitive markets.[30] In each case, there were incentives to cut back patient care to meet regulatory standards or to maintain competitive advantage.

HMO COMPETITION

Research on the impact of competition on HMOs is relatively varied and inconclusive, albeit somewhat less so than data for hospital competition.

The available studies looked at both the level of penetration and competition among HMOs in order to examine market effect, particularly focusing on quality and other nonprice variables. On the whole, the impact of competition was beneficial.

Positive Impact of HMO Competition

Rogowski and his colleagues examined the effect of increased HMO penetration in the health care market on hospital quality, measured by mortality rates for six medical conditions. The results were significant only for two of the six conditions, but for those two—gastrointestinal hemorrhage and congestive heart failure—as HMO penetration increased, mortality rates decreased.[31] Volpe and Buckley used data from 1989 through 1996 to examine the effect of increased HMO penetration on outcome and treatment patterns for acute myocardial infarctions. The results indicated that, as HMO penetration increased, the likelihood of receiving cardiac catheterization, angioplasty, or bypass surgery decreased by 3–16%, while rates of mortality remained constant. In a metropolitan statistical area, higher competition was modestly associated with a 2% increase in the rate of cardiac catheterizations.[32]

Another study found that, as the number of HMOs increased in a market, the premiums for health care consumers decreased. This effect was significant only for independent practice associations (IPAs) at the highest level of competition, but for group HMOs, this trend was noticeable at all levels of competition.[33] Mark et al. examined the effect of HMO penetration on the relationship between nursing staff and quality of care. Although the results did not indicate a statistically significant direct relationship between them, that data did show that, as HMO penetration increased, so did the number of registered nurses, which was associated with lower mortality rates and shorter lengths of stay.[34]

Negative and Neutral Impact of Competitive HMOs

There are also a number of studies which reveal that HMO penetration and competition is not associated with improvements in quality of care. Scanlon and his colleagues used data from 1999 to examine the effect of competition on HMOs operating in competitive and penetrated markets.

The results indicated no significant relationship between the level of market competition and HMO performance or quality of care. The authors also noted that their research led them to feel it necessary to re-evaluate the notion that market theory is beneficial for health care.[35]

Farasat Bokhari studied the relationship between market competition and the frequency of technology adoption. He found that an increase in competition among HMOs is positively correlated with the likelihood of a hospital adopting new technologies, mainly cardiac catheterization laboratories.[36] Additionally, Rivers and Fottler examined the impact of increased HMO competition and penetration on the quality of care provided, measured by risk-adjusted mortality rates. The study found no significant relationship among risk-adjusted mortality and HMO competition, penetration, and a combined measure of both. The author comments, "These results suggest that more intensely competitive markets, characterized by a high degree of managed care programs, may have no significant impact on quality of care."[37]

A COMPETITION MISCELLANY

I conclude, from my survey, that a number of efforts to assess competition in hospital and HMO competition were a draw, with evidence for and against. It is important to note, however, that most of the studies were mainly regional or local, which can be taken to mean that they offer few clues about national competition—or that they show that competitive success or failure is a matter of context.

I will conclude this section by moving beyond the hospital and HMO competition studies to comment on the FEHBP, and on a few other miscellaneous examples.

Federal Employees Health Benefit Program

FEHBP makes available to Federal employees a variety of health plan choices, with about twelve competitive plans available to all, and fifteen to twenty available to most of them. For a number of years, it has been offered as a model of consumer-directed and competitive health care by the market-inclined and was drawn upon as a model by some presidential candidates and others for their health care proposals.[38] As a kind of test case of a government program versus one rooted in the private sector, it has also been frequently compared with Medicare, with the latter found wanting by promarket advocates. Yet in some earlier years, Medicare had done better and in others the FEHBP, but the differences were marginal at best, alternating between an annual 5–6% cost increase a year between 2000 and 2003.

All of that has changed in the past few years. According to a 2007 paper prepared by the American Federation of Government Employees (AFGE) calling for overall program reform, average FEHBP premiums have risen by 60% over the past 7 years, an average of 8.5% a year, higher than the general average of the private sector of 7%, and the annual general rate of inflation of 2–3%.[39] Moreover, the government's portion of payment for the chosen program is declining as well while, at the same time, federal employees are seeing increased out-of-pocket costs, unpredictable shifts in covered benefits from year to year, and the sudden disappearance of popular plans.[40] A 2007 report by the Government Accountability Program noted that a study in that year of the ten largest insurance plans showed that they ranged from 0% to 15% in increased premiums, and together had ranged from a peak of 12.9% in 2002 to 1.8% in 2007. That low figure was, however, qualified by noting that it was the result of less generous coverage, enrollee migration to lower-cost plans, and withdrawals from a reserve fund. Had those changes not taken place, the 2007 increase would have been 9%. The FEHBP program does not pay the full insurance cost, but limits it to 72% of average premiums.[41] Those trends with FEHPB suggest that it is no longer a good example of effective competition, if indeed it ever had been. It now stands as a cautionary tale of a dependence upon the private sector to control costs.

COMMUNITY AND SPECIALTY HOSPITAL COMPETITION

Since the 1990s, specialty hospitals for a variety of conditions (psychiatric problems, cancer, heart conditions, and orthopedics, for example) have emerged, numbering over 100 by 2003. In that year, Congress established an 18-month moratorium on their further creation, alleging that they may constitute unfair and harmful competition with local community hospitals and that they also raise conflict-of-interest problems because most were started and owned by physicians.[42]

In March of 2005, the Medicare Payment Advisory Commission (MedPac) issued a report on the various competition and other issues, recommending an extension of the moratorium to January 1, 2007, after which the moratorium was dropped.[43] Their report, based on results through 2002, found that physician-owned specialty hospitals did not have lower costs for Medicare patients than those in community hospitals although patients did have shorter lengths of stay. The patients usually had less severe conditions, and there were fewer Medicaid patients in the specialty hospitals. Yet the community hospitals were effectively able to compete with the specialty hospitals, demonstrating comparable financial performance. The recommendation to extend the moratorium to 2007 was more the result of continuing worries about physician conflict-of-interest than about the economic effects of the competition.

If the FEHBP may now fail as an example of efficacious competition, specialty hospitals may succeed and not because of any proven economic superiority, but because it is now well recognized that patient health outcomes are generally superior in specialty facilities where repetition, patient numbers, and experience can lead to superior care.[44]

Assorted other examples of successful competition have been offered and should be mentioned.[45] The first set is that of cosmetic surgery, laser eye surgery, and generic drugs. The first two examples do not work well, however, because they are intensively advertised, not ordinarily covered by health insurance and for most patients (more properly called consumers in these cases), they are not "medically necessary" procedures in even the loosest definition of that term. Moreover, it might be added that if both procedures were covered by government or private insurance, their rapid growth in recent years would increase the aggregate costs for the plans and result in higher premiums for everyone. As the history of medical economics has shown, even if individual treatment costs decline, the pool of users typically increases and therewith the overall costs. Generic drugs are a better example, and they work well in favor of competition.

A different kind of example, interesting but a bit of a stretch, is the success of medical specialty units in a number of developing countries. They offer advanced surgery and other services at prices much lower than in the United States, and they attract a growing number of American patients. But most American patients are not likely to take their critical-care needs abroad nor are most American physicians likely to lower their fees to compete with professional colleagues in India, China, and Thailand. If that latter response should happen, that would surely put some points on the competition scoreboard. But apart from such an unlikely development, that kind of foreign competition is not very relevant to competition in America—but it could become so, depending upon how far the off-shore possibilities develop. Then we would see if subspecialty physicians (especially surgeons) would reduce their (usually) high fees to meet the competition.

EUROPEAN HEALTH CARE AND THE MOVE
TO AN EXPANSION OF COMPETITION

Before moving on to the last phases of my examination of competition, it is interesting to take a side look at European competition initiatives. Market initiatives in European health care, of which there are many, are unfamiliar to most Americans. If the American scene is confusing—a mixture of no evidence where some would be relevant, and of mixed results where some evidence is available—the European landscape is no less so. The market in general and competition in particular have attracted much European attention over at least the past three decades. In great part that has happened because of increased economic pressures on health care, rising political resistance to government control (although not as intense as in the United States), and the stirring of consumer-directed interests. At the same time, it is important to note that competition is less advanced in Europe, with few empirical studies.

But there are some intriguing features of the European developments that should be of interest to Americans. The first is that, because of the economic pressures on their health care systems, Europeans are looking in a market direction despite an historical resistance to doing so; and they are looking to the United States for some models, a striking move for countries that have traditionally been scornful of American health care.

The second is that the European countries have struggled with the problem of how to maintain universal care while at the same time introducing competition and other market efforts. They perceive a fundamental tension in comingling the two, attractive because of possible economic and other benefits, but threatening as well because such merging introduces values at odds with those that have traditionally sustained their systems, most notably solidarity and equal access. The main U.S. debate on health care reform is how to develop a good government–market balance, and the European experience offers an important way to go about this.

The Dutch health analyst Frederick D. Schut and his colleagues at Rotterdam University have noted three phases in recent European health care: a first wave of universal coverage and equal access; a second wave of controls, rationing and spending caps; and the present third wave, the use of market incentives and competition.[46] But it is no less clear that this third wave is in severe tension with a commitment to the strong and persistent role of government, especially of regulation, as a political commitment and reality. The European response to that tension has been to see the market as complementing government control, using it to strengthen solidarity and universal care, not to compete with it. That has been a delicate and difficult task, if only because European traditions and government power, not readily relinquished, stand directly in the path of market freedom. The nations of Europe understandably want both, a familiar human and political problem that sometimes succeeds and sometimes does not.

I first consider two European countries that have actively and perhaps most prominently pursued increased competition and then present some more general reflections on the European scene by a variety of commentators. The two countries are The Netherlands and the United Kingdom, although Germany, Belgium, and Sweden have initiated various competition efforts as well, as have most other countries to a lesser degree.[47]

The Netherlands

As a small nation with few natural resources, The Netherlands has had to live as a nation of traders, by its market wits. In many ways even more than the United States, it has a deep pragmatic-libertarian strain, reflecting an uncommonly strong devotion to individual liberty. Its acceptance of some narcotics, legal prostitution, and euthanasia testify to that national strain. It has also a deep commitment to solidarity and universal care. Its culture, then, is more than most European countries open to market values, and The Netherlands is aggressively trying to embody these in its universal health care system.

Although the Dutch explored competitive practices in recent years, 2006 marked the introduction of stronger and more systematic efforts, which the government calls "managed competition," the language at least obviously influenced by Alain Enthoven's pioneering work.[48] Its new policy allows everyone to switch insurers once a year; requires insurers to compete with each other based on a packet of benefits determined by government; permits deductibles and competitive premiums; allows insurers to buy health care from providers for their clients; permits providers to compete with each other and to sell health care services to insurers; and takes advantage of the fact that a strong majority of hospitals and other care providers are private. At the same time, the new policy reinforces solidarity and universality by embodying many limits to consumer choice and provider behavior.

There have been some early results reported. In 2006 some 19% of the insured switched to another insurer, and one insurer was driven out of business. Premiums were lower than expected, but there was evidently a strong effort by insurers to increase their market share with low rates, and most of them did not cover an increase in their expenditures. As a compensatory catch-up move, premium costs were expected to rise by 8–10% in 2007. The Dutch government does not control the premium rates of insurers. Another effect of consumer competition has been to stimulate more consolidations, and three consortiums of insurers now cover close to 75% of the market. Price competition in the hospital sector is, however, controlled, but with some recent modifications. Prices can be freely negotiated for 20% of total expenditures, an increase from an earlier 10%. The Minister of Health has said the aim is to extend the scope of that market freedom but how far is not clear. One seasoned observer, noting a cautious implementation process, believes that the government will not go so far as to lose control of expenditures.[49]

It is probably too early to judge the long-term success of the new policy, but it has been put in place with strong enough government support to give it a good chance of increasing the scope and impact of competition. Just what difference that will make to cost control, quality, and efficiency remains unclear, if only because the commitment to solidarity and government regulation will inevitably weaken market freedom. The evidence to date, however, is less than positive. As two analysts have concluded, the first two years of the 2006 reforms show that the "new Dutch model may not control costs. . . . consumer [insurance] premiums are increasing . . . public satisfaction is not high, and perceived quality is down."[50] The Dutch policy, moreover, has not been based on prior evidence of likely success or on market experiments in health care. It represents what one leading Dutch policy analyst, Hans Maarse, calls an ideological paradigm shift in Dutch social policy, with competition as a key element in health care as well as elsewhere. "The Dutch government," he has written, "assumes that it is possible to achieve public ends with private means if only competition is well regulated."[51] The Dutch government, he says, aims for a price–quality competition. An open question is whether price competition will weaken quality competition, a familiar issue in competition studies.

The United Kingdom

In the United Kingdom, an interest in the market and health care first came strongly to the fore during the Margaret Thatcher administration from 1979–1997, which saw a shift from an earlier welfare state consensus to an advocacy of markets to meet social needs and to diminish the power of government. Yet in comparison with the privatization of the railroads and the postal service, the National Health Services came out relatively unscathed, a tribute to its popularity. Tax breaks were provided for private health insurance and what came to be called "internal markets" were developed, allowing for greater provider choice and competition. What also began to develop was what Alan Cribb of Kings College London has called a managerial mode of organization, a move away from a bureaucratic model.

Little power to regulate health care was taken from the government in the Thatcher era, however, and those market moves had little impact. The advent of Tony Blair and the Labour government in 1998 sought a "third way" between a liberal social democracy and a conservative New Right as a general policy, and with it, a "second wave" of health care reforms. While the language of markets and competition was put into the background, replaced with the softer terminology of partnership and collaboration, the internal market approach remained in place and with a greater degree of private sector involvement. Providers have been pushed by the government to compete with each other on quality but not on price, which remains to this day under considerable government control.

As in The Netherlands, there is a worry among Labour Party members that the market initiatives will subvert the long-standing universal care commitment; and complaints have been rising about the increasingly abusive use of NHS facilities by physicians working primarily in the private sector. The embrace of competition has been weakly supported by analogies to other market activities within the purview of government, but the main drive has come from a combination of ideology and a belief in the efficiency that the market moves will introduce. Evidence in favor of competition in health care has not been directly introduced as an argument in its favor: little has been offered, and little seems available. There is a recognition, as in The Netherlands, that competition and heavy regulation do not make for a good partnership, but they still want to try for it.

This brief focus on two countries only—but ones that have some of the most vigorous debate and attention to health care—is surely inadequate to draw any decisive conclusions on the impact of competition policies more generally. But I was unable to turn up any good information anywhere about whether empirical evidence is adduced to initiate competition efforts or gathered to demonstrate its efficacy once in place. Cost control has in most countries been pursued by price controls and various forms of government-dominated regulation rather than by competition. And competition efforts have focused more on quality of care and efficiency than price control.

European competition efforts seem to have succeeded best in giving patients more choice. Competition on both price and quality among insurers and other providers has been restricted because of regulation, a dilemma earlier noted, but more with the former than with the latter. Jost and his colleagues conclude that "the evidence indicates that European instruments for controlling costs [regulation primarily] have been more effective than the U.S. reliance on competition."[52]

COMPETITION: THE FIX THAT WILL FAIL

What does my survey of various American and European competitive efforts reveal? I judge them to be mixed and inconclusive, particularly the American initiatives where there has been more actual and evaluated competition. Sometimes competition works, and sometimes it does not. Sometimes it works for quality improvement but not cost control and sometimes it does not; and sometimes it works for costs but not quality. There are no good reasons, based on evidence, to think it can work on a national scale to control costs.

Like many American advocates of competition, Europeans are willing to put it in place without insisting on prior empirical evidence in support of doing so, heavily influenced by business, rather than health care, evidence. They seem so far to have carried out little research to determine if it is working where it is already in place. Even where there is some evidence, in the United States and Europe, that competition in some local circumstances can help control costs and improve quality, the benefits are usually marginal.

In any case, the American situation shows what scientists might call a "natural experiment," that is one that has not been organized as an experiment but simply developed on its own. That experiment shows that, for over 30 years, competition in the private sector, particularly among insurers, has simply and flatly failed to stop a steady annual cost inflation well beyond the annual growth of GDP. Hospitals still use technology, the latest and the best if they can afford it, to compete with each other, and everyone seems to want more, not less, technology. Insurers cannot dodge the technology bullet any better than anyone else.

In a detailed empirical examination of competition in American health care from 1993–2005, Joseph White concluded that

> . . . market forces are unlikely to improve costs and access, compared with the methods used in other countries. First [if the aim is universal access it] depends on some people subsidizing others, and markets are no in the business of creating subsidies . . . Second, cost control must begin with limiting prices . . . the evidence from the American health care market since 1993 suggests that prices were the primary variable in cost control performance . . . effective reform will require restraining the market, not relying on it.[53]

White has assessed costs with a thoroughness well beyond what supporters of competition have done. The cumulative data from his research and that of others show that the private sector has not done as well as

TABLE 1
Percentage Increase in Health Care Costs per Capita, United States, 1970–2004

Years	All Benefits[a]		Common Benefits[b]		GDP per Capita
	Medicare	PHI[c]	Medicare	PHI	
1970–2004	9.2	10.9	8.9	9.9	6.1
1970–1993	10.9	12.8	10.7	12.0	7.1
1993–1997	7.6	4.3	6.4	2.6	4.3
1997–1999	−0.2	5.9	1.4	4.3	4.3
1999–2004	6.4	9.5	5.8	8.6	3.7

[a] "All Benefits" refers to total costs for Medicare and private insurance.
[b] "Common Benefits" refers to costs for services covered by both Medicare and private insurance plans. For example, "Common Benefits" excludes most prescription drug costs.
[c] PHI = Private Health Insurance.
Source: Costs are from Centers for Medicare and Medicaid Services, National Health Expenditure Data, table 13, http://www.cms.hhs.gov/NationalHealthExpendData/downloads/tables.pdf (accessed June 18, 2007).
GDP is from 2006 Economic Report of the President, table B-31, http://a257.g.akamaitech.net/7/257/2422/15feb20061000/www.gpoaccess.gov/eop/2006/B31.xls (accessed June 18, 2007).
Reprinted from Joseph White, "Markets and Medical Care: The United States, 1993–2005," The Milbank Quarterly 85, no. 3 (2007): 405.

Medicare in controlling costs, and that it is a weak reed to lean on. Table 1 displays that evidence.

There is a response to unfavorable evidence among the market-oriented. Few success stories of competition in health care are offered. The reigning models of competition benefits are drawn from the business sector. Health care competition in the United States has failed, it is said, because it is either misdirected or badly stifled by government regulation; real competition has not been allowed to work.[54] A spate of market-oriented books in 2005–2006 gave competition a central role in health reform, but the emphasis (with a couple of exceptions) was on the allegedly deadening effect of regulation. "The balance of evidence," two analysts wrote in The Business of Health, "suggests that markets have much to offer, and the unencumbered functioning of health care markets has largely been untested in the United States."[55] With the exception of medical specialty hospitals, which do show some competitive advantages, their other examples of competition, health insurance and pharmaceuticals, are used to talk about regulatory burdens on competition, but with no offered evidence of the cost control potential.

In another book, *Healthy Competition*, the authors contend that "consumers who are free to choose from competing options and who face tradeoffs among competing options [are among conditions that] . . . actually promote lower prices and higher quality."[56] Little evidence is offered to support that statement, and the emphasis of the book falls on pursuing the deregulation of competition. Greater physician freedom for the use of off-label prescription drugs and a loosening of FDA regulations are the examples given of how to manage technology costs.[57]

The authors of a third book, *Healthy, Wealthy, & Wise*, propose "greater federal scrutiny of anticompetitive behavior by hospitals and other healthcare providers . . . "[58] "Markets," they concede, "will not eliminate growth in health care costs—an inevitable product of technological change . . . or how to finance care for the low-income chronically ill. But the power of markets to allocate resources efficiently—power evident in every other sector of the economy—is part of the solution."[59] That is a modest enough conclusion and different from faith in the market evident in the other two books; but even for this contention they offer little direct evidence from the medical sector. That it may work in other sectors of the economy does not prove it will work equally well in health care (and it hardly works that way all the time in the private sector).

In sum, the argument of these three books is that a reduction of regulation will enhance competition and let the market work its magic. Yet whether deregulation will deliver better results is speculative and hypothetical; maybe so and maybe not—and whether deregulation could politically even be put into place on a large scale is speculative as well. An impressive example of this phenomenon is a large and elaborately argued book by Michael Porter and Elizabeth Olmsted Teisberg. They press for new modes of competition (competition for value and results not what they call the present cost-shifting form), but it is so complex that it is hard to imagine it making its way through Congress.[60] It offers little in the way of hard evidence from health care to support its idealized goals. Nor does it deal with the relativity of value as noted above or its enormously varied meaning for individuals. A colleague in The Netherlands has told me that their book has been influential there, although the Dutch moves toward more competition do not sound like anything presented in their book.[61]

THE COMPETITION: CANADIAN
AND EUROPEAN HEALTH CARE

But with what is competition (and other market practices) being compared? What is competition competing with? Typically it has been Canadian and European health care, cited for its bureaucracy, its government regulation, its stifling of technological innovation, its control of medical practice, and its lack of consumer choice. The United States, it is frequently said, has the best health care in the world; and that fact helps explain, so it is said, why so many foreigners come here for specialized care. It is no less the case, the argument goes, that the United States is the leader in Nobel prizes for medicine and biology, the world's leading source of pharmaceutical and device innovation, and for those with good insurance coverage a surpassingly high level of medical care. Yes, we have our problems, but they are correctible, and in any event our strengths, warts and all, are superior to those of government-run health care systems.

That overall judgment is inaccurate. At the least, it most commonly ignores the great variety of universal care systems. They are as different from each other as Denmark is culturally different from Italy, Norway from France. The usual starting point for criticisms of those systems is that of the United Kingdom and Canada, and particularly their notorious waiting lists, as if their experience tells the whole story of government-controlled systems. But their experience does not even come close. As it happens, those two countries rank very low on comparative studies of developed countries, close to the bottom (along with the United States).

France, generally ranked the best, with no waiting lists of any consequence, hardly gets a mention. Ironically, international surveys have consistently shown a number of Scandinavian countries, famous for their welfare systems, to be at the top of the international list (together with the United States) of countries with the most competitive economies. European efforts to use competition in the service of universal care (not to compete with it) are rarely noted or acknowledged.

The available and historically consistent international evidence supports the superiority of European health care in just about every relevant category of cost, quality, access, and popularity.[62] If the competition between the market and government were based on comparative evidence, the United States would be a clear loser.

Why then is the evidence, hardly hidden, ignored or minimized? One answer is the obvious and long-standing American resistance to a government-dominated system (save for Medicare, Medicaid, the Veterans Administration, and assorted smaller programs, now close of 50% of our health care); like it or not, many believe, it is not going to happen here, and should not happen here, evidence or not. One is reminded of the old joke about the child who does not like carrots: "I don't like carrots, and if I tasted them I might like them, but I don't like them." Yet the drift toward a larger government role and the popularity of Medicare and the Veterans Administration programs may display more acceptance of government than the standard stereotype has it.

The other reason for resistance may be that the English-speaking countries, our cultural cousins, are taken to be the pertinent comparisons, as if those countries across the channel are disqualified from comparisons. But the United Kingdom and Canada have tax-based (Beveridge) systems, with direct government control, financial and managerial; and they work less well than the systems of the continental countries. The latter have many Social Health Insurance systems (e.g. France, Switzerland, The Netherlands). They are paid for by mandated employee-employer contributions working with quasi-independent insurance agencies; and they offer patients as wide a range of choices as that of any American patient. They are a more pertinent model for American emulation—with many varieties to choose from—and are in most respects superior to, but also slightly more expensive than, the tax-based systems.

TESTING COMPETITION

Cost control has long been a preoccupation in American health care, going back at least to the Nixon administration in 1970. Competition has for an equally long time been proposed as an important antidote. "We can't go on like this" has been the persistent lament, year after year, decade after decade, and any number of cost-control strategies have been tried. None have made much difference save for a short period in the mid-1990s when HMOs did two things. They imposed a number of requirements, but patient and physician resistance to them brought that phase to an end, and insurers could not sustain low premiums. Costs once again headed up. If the evidence in favor of competition is inadequate to justify giving it a central place in American health care reform, what are some options for giving it a role? Five of them can be imagined.

Unregulated Competition

The first possibility would simply be to take a chance on unregulated competition, working to improve it qua effective competition, but not to regulate or control its cost outcomes. Any form of serious and comprehensive American health reform will be a gamble, and one might argue that unfettered competition is at least a decent bet and should be given a chance of succeeding. That argument would not be persuasive, given the weak likelihood of the gamble paying off. The fact that this model *might* work is not good enough. Its failure would wreck the system as costs continued to escalate beyond any sensible point of sustainability. Even a little success would not show it capable of comprehensively cutting costs to the extent necessary.

Competition with Fallback Regulation

A second possibility would be to pursue competition, working also to improve it, but with a proviso: if after 3 to 4 years competition began failing significantly to reduce annual cost increases, then the government would be empowered to step in and impose an annual limit on cost escalation, such as on drug prices and insurance premiums. That would also be a gamble, but one with a kind of bettor's ceiling, limiting the harmful effects of a no-limit gamble. It would also allow competition supporters a chance to test their convictions but with the understanding that they would pay a decisive penalty if their system failed.

Competition with Regulation

A third possibility would be to build in cost escalation limits on private competition right from the start. That might be done with a staggered series of benchmarks: to reduce annual cost increases from 7% at present to 6% 2 years later, to 5% in another 2 years, and then to 4% in an additional 2 years. This method would create an even stronger incentive than the first one, making it utterly clear that a reduction of cost escalation was not just a pious hope or a fine ideal, but an absolute short-term necessity.

COMPETITION WITHIN A PUBLIC CHOICE PLAN

President Obama, Senator Max Baucus, and and former Senator Tom Daschle, have all proposed a public insurance option for those who do not have employer-based health coverage. The political scientist Jacob S. Hacker has laid out the case for such an option greater detail than they have provided—called the Public Plan Choice—and I will draw upon his account.[63]

The Plan would be managed by the federal government but with the medical care tendered by private providers. It would be offered through a national insurance "exchange," and that exchange would compete with private insurance coverage. The premise of the plan is that public insurance, notably Medicare, has done much better at reining in costs than private insurance, and thus should serve as a benchmark for the private sector. Medicare has seen a 4.6% growth in costs between 1997 and 2006 compared with 7.3% for private insurance, and it has been estimated by the Lewin Group that a plan along the Public Choice line could save $1000 a year on coverage. Given that advantage it makes sense to use it as a standard "against which private plans must compete. Without a public plan . . . we will continue to lack strong mechanisms to rein in costs and drive value down the road."

A key provision is that, while the Public Choice Plan would serve as a benchmark, "the public and private plans must compete side by side on a level playing field." Each would have to offer a comparable package of benefits, the private plans would have to accept all applicants, and there would be no limitation of coverage based on preexisting conditions. Underlying the concept of competing public and a private coverage is the assumption, based on public opinion surveys, that the public would prefer such a mix, not one oriented too heavily in a government or private direction.

I have three reservations. First, it is not clear what a "level playing field" means if the federal public program would have a $1000 cost advantage while offering the same package of benefits as the private pro-

viders. Why would anyone want a private plan under those circumstances? Or is it that the latter would have to compete by offering, at a
higher price, a wider range of coverage and higher quality of some kind?
No answers to those questions are discernible. In any case, is it politically
likely that the private insurers would tolerate a competition which pos-
ited them as the likely losers? They can run the numbers as well as
anyone else.

Second, the competition would be limited to those "who lack
employment-based insurance." Since that would only be some 15% of
the population, its impact on the overall cost of health care, the other
85%, would be minimal. Only if available to everyone as, say, an option
open to those covered by their employers would it make a great difference to overall health care costs.

Third, there is nothing in the plan outside of the limited Public Choice
competition that would force the private sector to change its characteristic commercial behavior. They would be free to set prices as they now
do, with the well-known historical result that those prices, whether for
insurance premiums or drug prices, would continue to rise unabated.
Fourth, even the 4.6% annual cost growth figure for Medicare is too
great, by at least 50%, in terms of the long-term need for parity with
the annual increase of the GDP. And if the 7.3% annual increase in the
private sector remains at that level, then the net result is that the restricted range of the Public Choice Plan will make little long term difference to the more broadly based cost escalation.

UNIVERSAL CARE

A fifth possibility would be to move far more decisively in a government-
managed direction. Such a move need not necessarily be to a single
payer, tax-based reform plan (the weaknesses of which can be seen in
Canadian and British health care), but to one more along the lines of
European Social Health Insurance. Through employer–employee mandated coverage, supplemented by government subsidies for the elderly,
the unemployed, and others outside the employment market, coverage
would be universal. But it could, as in Switzerland and The Netherlands,
be provided by private but strongly regulated health care insurers who
are forced to live with limits to cost escalation.

The advantage of that last possibility is that, as it does in Europe, regulation would work to control costs far more effectively than is now possible in the United States. Unlike our present situation, a government-managed and -regulated health care system could draw upon a variety of sources for ideas and ongoing experiments. These would include the following sources: (1) the European efforts to use competition to strengthen universal care by the use of competition, not to compete with it; and the European goal in many countries of working out a good balance between competition and government regulation of that competition; (2) the Medicare, VA, and Medicaid programs, which have many good features, and with a wide range of reform experiments underway. Most notably these programs have controlled costs far better than the private sector has—but still not enough. One reason the cuts have not been enough is that these programs are still within the fee-for-service model, heavily influenced by the private sector, on which they are heavily dependent. That can be changed. We must keep in mind the success of HMOs in controlling costs in the mid-1990s. They were an economic success and a political failure; but political failures are reversible in different times under different circumstances.

My organization, The Hastings Center, with 32 employees, provides health care insurance for everyone. Over the pat three years we have used three different insurers: Aetna, Oxford, and Empire Bluecross Blueshield. They compete with each other for our business, and we have changed each year based on close, and changing, votes by the staff. Their annual premiums are within less than $1000 of each other (in the $13,500 range for family coverage) and the only noticeable differences among them are on copayments and deductibles and out-of-network coverage; and they fluctuate each year, but also within a close range of each other. Our Empire premium rose by 15% in 2009, and their competitors would have done the same. It seems self-evident that "competition" of that kind makes no significant contribution to controlling national costs.

A regulation-free, unfettered competition offers no reasonable possibility of controlling costs. The attraction of technology for patients and physicians, abetted by energetic and relentless industry marketing, has shown itself capable of overwhelming the private sector's control efforts, driving up costs despite competition. The fact that successful competitive strategies require finding ingenious ways of competing simultaneously on quality and price, for which no ideal solution has ever been found, is part of the problem. As a long-time reader of *Consumer Reports*, I find it interesting that many poorly evaluated products continue to sell, even turning a profit for their manufacturers. They may lose market share, but that does not mean they will not be bought. Could not the same thing happen in a CDHC with competitive providers and insurers with large numbers of people, despite good information on the range of available choices not making good choices about their health plan? Why not?

It would be reckless to depend upon competition to control costs and technology, especially in a model that could not easily be reversed if it failed. If that judgment is reasonable given the available evidence, then the choice before the country is a stark one: either be prepared to regulate health care costs and prices, or accept the continuing decline of employer-provided health care dependent on private insurers. The former trend would make countless interest groups and market-oriented interest groups unhappy in countless ways, but the control of costs would offer the public some needed relief. The latter trend would lead to the dominance and growth of a private sector that would offer more and more competitive choices, the good ones all but unaffordable (save for the affluent), and the poor ones all but useless (for the rest of us).

CHAPTER 5

THE COHABITATION OF
MEDICINE AND COMMERCE

Earlier chapters in this book could well have given the impression that technology is somehow an independent actor with a life of its own. This is not so, even though the cultural force of a commitment to technological innovation is an important part of the story. Technology costs are determined by those who invent it, prescribe it, and consume it, and the relationship between medicine and industry is the central part of that combination.

If a love of medical technology is deeply rooted in an American culture long enamored of all forms of technology, a love of commerce is easily competitive. The two have become comfortable partners based on a complex relationship among science, the government, private industry, and the medical profession. The federal government provides much of the basic research that opens the door for clinical applications, industry translates that research into those applications, and then sells them to the public through the conduit of physicians. At the end of that chain are patients, not only beholden to doctors in gaining prescriptions and treatments, but of late the recipients of industry media advertisements and internet information.

Those interconnections make the control of technology costs exceedingly difficult, and the carrots for the use of technology far exceed any disincentives for its use. There are few sticks to use because each of the actors, from industry through medicine through patients, has a vested interest in the enterprise. Their shields are easily able to ward off the sticks. Were it not for the cost problem, the medical technology industry would be basking in unblemished popularity. Yet despite years of attacks, that industry has been successful in turning the cost problem on its head, linking its high prices directly to its great benefits, a fine exemplar of the market in action. Medicine, for its part, has organized its educational system and its working culture into a commitment to use technology as its main weapon again illness, suffering, and death. Patients have responded in kind, far more drawn to the technologies that can save and improve their lives when they are sick than to the more tedious efforts necessary to prevent illness in the first place. Congress has over the years blessed the entire enterprise, protecting it from serious cost controls and orienting the Medicare program in the direction of technology consumption.

Is there a way to break into those interconnections, tightly bound together, to make better use of technology and to reduce its costs? Not easily. One reason is that there are many links to be dealt with, not one of which can be managed without changing the others. The contention of this chapter is that the technology industry is the important link, the one most influential in shaping the others. Physicians have their own traditions and culture but ones that are intertwined with industry. For patients, there is no way that industry can be avoided. They are being cared for by physicians who use its products and deluged by a flood of advertisements and publicity in favor of them. Congress, sensitive to political pressures, public opinion, and a flock of lobbyists wants to help, not hinder, industry and goes out of its way to do so.

The industry draws its greatest strength from the deep national commitment—one shaped by our history, culture, and politics—to the market as an enhancer of individual freedom and the main engine of economic growth and prosperity. Although there is no doubt that the large amount of money the industry invests in political contributions gives it a leg up with Congress, that underlying cultural base gives it an added edge. The practical fact of the matter is that, despite long-standing complaints about its prices and its political influence, the power of supply and demand trumps the gnashing of teeth. However high the costs or sharp the criticism of industry, the public has shown it will buy its products. Undeterred by criticism, the industry simply raises its prices to ever higher levels and plunges ahead, reaping the highest profit of any industry. Why would they not, given that very nice bottom line? A Yale coach many years ago, with a constantly losing football team, said of the alumni that "they should be kept sullen, but not mutinous." The technology industry walks that line brilliantly.

ILL-FATED TECHNOLOGY ASSESSMENT EFFORTS

At bottom, the industry does two things: it vigorously markets its products, and it no less vigorously stands in the way of any all efforts to curtail its market freedom. A most useful cautionary care, and a good way into the industry role, is the story of the demise of the National Center for Health Care Technology, established by Congress in 1978 and dying an unnatural death in 1981 when Congress would not renew its support. It was shot down by opposition from the American Medical Association and the Health Industry Manufacturers Association. Because there has been much talk in recent years about establishing a technology assessment program, the history of this agency is eerily disturbing. As the author of that story, Seymour Perry—whose article is a fine and revealing analysis on the agency's demise—noted at the time, some 25 years ago, "it is likely that similar objections will be raised against any future efforts to reinstitute a formal mechanism for assessing medical technology, whether in the government or the private sector."[1] (Conservative commentators on the $1.1 billion for technology assessment in the Obama stimulus package did indeed press "similar objections.")

The aim of the National Center was to assess medical technology for its safety, efficacy, economics, ethics and impact on society. It was, Perry writes, "a unique, unprecedented effort to establish in the executive branch of government a formal and neutral mechanism for providing assessments of health-care technologies to policy-makers, the Medicare program, the medical profession, and others."[2] It was not, however, given a regulatory or cost-containment role, although the inclusion of safety and economics within its scope of analysis implicitly opened the door to them. Yet if the agency itself was a part of government, "its philosophy was that the private sector, not the federal bureaucracy, was the appropriate place for the assessment of technologies."[3] It was meant to be neutral in its work, serving mainly as an initiator and catalyst. An important part of that role was support of extramural grants, some 50% of its budget, for original research, evaluations of specific technologies, and demonstrations.

Technologies were divided into three categories: emerging technologies (not yet undergoing clinical trials), new technologies (but not widely disseminated), and old or existing technologies. Its work with Medicare was to develop evaluation criteria for the safety and clinical effectiveness of technologies for coverage recommendations, although in line with Medicare's exclusion from cost implications—"necessary and reasonable" only—it could not go near that problem. Despite a few restrictions and limitations, the National Center had "the support and cooperation of virtually every medical-specialty society and of large umbrella organizations in the health-technology industry."[4]

None of that support, or its neutral role regarding medical technology, was enough to keep the Center alive. Despite apparent support in principle by the Reagan administration—which had earlier actually called for such an agency, "one designed to screen procedures . . . [and to provide a mechanism] that would not deny the right to perform disputed procedures, only to announce that Medicare and Medicaid . . . would not pay for them"—the opposition of the AMA and the Health Industry Manufacturers Association was too much to bear. The AMA was worried that the program would interfere with the practice of medicine, which had traditionally taken care of "risks and costs, as well as benefits . . . as central to the exercise of good medical judgment."[5] In other words, it remained up to individual doctors to continue making such judgments as they always had, since the days of Hippocrates, free of government intervention, even of the softest kind.

The Manufacturers Association said that the Center was not needed and that technology assessment was already under way in some twenty agencies, an argument that Perry rejected by out of hand, noting that the claim was valid "only to the extent that health was an interest to all," and none of which had a mandate comparable to the Center. Hovering over the debate was the familiar primordial fear that the Center "would stifle innovation." Both that fear as well as a threat to the independence of physicians in treating patients, have of course had a hardy and resilient shelf life in the 27 years since then.

Although its program was not quite killed by Congress, the Agency for Health Care Policy and Research (AHCPR), whose 1985 charter was similar in many ways to the earlier National Center, was another effort at assessment, broader in its scope than the National Center. But it suffered, as Shannon Brownlee nicely put it, a "near death" in 1994. Its budget was cut, it was renamed the Agency for Health Care Quality and Research, and it was stripped of its power to recommend payment decisions to Medicaid and Medicare. AHCPR's undoing was to run afoul of back surgeons who were outraged at its recommendation of nonsurgical treatments.[6] While most of its work was focused on a wide range of technologies (including some projects on medical technology), the demise of a third agency, the Office of Technology Assessment (1974–1995), was just one more sign of Congressional resistance to the threat of assessment. Almost all of the reform proposals talked of establishing an assessment agency as well, but any such idea would have to go through Congress, obviously not a certain friend of such a move.

MASTERS OF POLITICAL CLOUT: THE MEDICAL INDUSTRY

There are at least three major medical industries that, taken together, have considerable economic and political power. Each has a powerful professional and lobbying organization. They are the Pharmaceutical Research and Manufacturers of America (PhRMA), Advanced Medical Technology Association (AdvaMed), and the Biotechnology Industry Organization (BIO). There are a number of smaller ones, but those three are the major actors. Taken together, their industries provide millions of American jobs, spend billions of dollars in local communities, are fine stock market investments, and make billions in sales to the domestic and international market.

Although subject to some federal and state regulations, mainly on safety, those industries are fine examples of the market in practice. They spend large amounts of money on research, still larger amounts on marketing their products, and they have managed to keep the government and cost-cutters at bay. They have powerful lobbies in Congress—spending about $1 billion in the past decade alone—and an enormous amount of economic clout to support all this. They have very effectively stopped dead in its tracks any effort to control their prices. PhRMA effectively blocked Medicare's ability to negotiate pharmaceutical prices with drug companies, although the VA has been able to do so for decades. The medical device industry is thought to be heavily responsible for the unwillingness of Congress to take account of costs in its Medicare benefit decisions. The pharmaceutical industry has effectively blocked drug importation from Canada and won for itself with the MMA the advantage of government subsidies for HMOs, private insurers, and corporations to purchase drugs.[7] The biotechnology industry has managed to market some extraordinarily expensive products despite some internal and public debates about doing so.

The most common argument the industry makes in support of its high prices is not only that it provides great health benefits, but that its profits and prices are necessary to continue creative research and innovation and, thus, to save future lives. While there has been dispute about how much its research actually costs (the drug companies say $800 million to bring a new drug to market) and how much it spends to market its products (more than it spends on research), the power of their innovation argument seems to be most effective with Congress and the public. As noted in earlier chapters, even many of those who agree that technology costs are the greatest problem in controlling health costs often blanche, and back down, at that thought that innovation might be stifled. They emphasize instead ridding ourselves of useless and wasteful treatments and technologies rather than confronting the useful and expensive ones. It seems assumed that any and all technology costs, as long as they can show some therapeutic benefit, ought to be considered acceptable and worth paying for.

Three questions can be asked about the emphasis on endless innovation. The first is why the future lives that will be improved or saved from a steady stream of innovations are more important than the lives that could now be saved if prices were lower. I have never seen the industry address that question at all, but I suppose it would be hard to come up with a good answer if it did. It was certainly a question implicit in the debate over the high cost of treatments for HIV disease, particularly in developing countries. Future victims of future diseases could hardly be worse off than present victims of that present scourge.[8] Only the greatest of international pressure forced the industry to back down in the HIV case to some extent, and then only abroad, less so in the United States.

The second question relates to a point I will develop in chapter 5. Just how much better health do we need as a society, and where ought the priorities lie? While the medical industry makes much of its contribution to national health, its prime focus is on individual health, as its disease-focused advertisements emphasize. It is not in the business of improving public or population health but of responding to individual preferences and needs. That response is a black hole, where nothing that is good enough today to satisfy patients will be good enough tomorrow, and where the newest drug or device is usually thought preferable to older ones, even if the evidence shows that is not so. But then there is a nice convergence for industry: it needs to innovate to keep making profits and growing, and patients (and their doctors) believe that innovation is the key to their future health.

Here is a piece of research that someone with appropriate credentials might carry out. If, say, innovation had stopped dead 10 years ago, but that everyone received at that time and since then the best treatment of that era for whatever their medical problems, what would have been the population health impact? My guess is that it would be at least as good as in our present situation and perhaps better by virtue of universal coverage of everyone. At the least, many conditions inadequately treated then, but for which good treatments existed, would have become available to everyone (e.g., hypertension treatment). I do not suppose industry would be a good candidate to support such a research project, and even the NIH, devoted to industry and innovation, might not be too enthused either. The whole point of such an exercise would not be to stop innovation but, instead, to determine just how much it actually improves health. The fact that costs continue to rise at a pace far greater than any decrease in morbidity and mortality provides a clue. But if we could have a better sense about what level of available technology and innovation makes a health difference, a base for resistance to industry and sensible priorities would be available

A third question might be this: even if we agreed that endless innovation for any and all medical ills, or to serve all desires and preferences, is not needed, will not research be necessary to avoid a decline in population health? We know, for instance, that antibiotic resistance is growing, that infectious disease kills people as much now as 30 to 40 years ago, and that new diseases continue to emerge, such as HIV disease. We know that obesity is increasing and will have growing deleterious effects in the future. I believe that newly emergent threats are an important area for research and innovation. They offer a different reason for innovation than the most common one, that individuals are still getting sick and dying, heavily from diseases of aging. It is true that they are, but no amount of technological innovation will put an end to that; the causes of death just get moved around a bit.

WARDING OFF CRITICISM

Over the years, the pharmaceutical industry has, among the others, come under the harshest criticism. The list of complaints is long, and, because they are now familiar, I will not rehash them at length here. They include (1) the creation of "me too" drugs, that is, drugs with little if any improvement over earlier-developed ones to provide the same treatment (and the industry even successfully persuaded the government to let new drugs be compared only with placebos rather than existing drugs, making it much harder to prove their value); (2) the permission to use direct-to-consumer advertising, a tactic rejected by every other country in the world save for New Zealand (and the industry expected, as happened, that a majority of physicians would most likely go along with patient requests as long as the requested drug would do no harm; why fight with patients?); (3) pursuit of physicians to prescribe their drugs, or think favorably about their companies, by every possible means, fair or foul including free meals, lavish trips to medical conferences, generous honoraria for lecturing on their products, trinkets, free tickets to sporting events, and free samples of drugs . . . on and on; (4) campaign contributions for members of Congress, the placement of former pharmaceutical company executives in federal regulatory agencies, issue ads on matters favorable toward the industry, and the employment as lobbyists of many former, and well-known, Congressmen (Connie Mack, Birch Bayh, and Dennis DiConcini); (5) extensive lobbying efforts in many useful directions—during the 2003–2004 election year, the industry spent $150 million to influence Congress and the public including $73 million at the federal level (mainly directed at Congress), $5 million to lobby the FDA, $49 million for advocacy at the state level, and $18 million to fight price controls and to protect patent rights abroad;[9] (6) paying providers to use drugs; (7) purchase of generic drug companies to help continue the sale of older, name brand drugs.[10]

Medicalization

Perhaps the most telling impact of industry and other efforts to make us pay attention to our health is that of persuading us that (1) we might already be at risk for illness and not know it (hypertension), or (2) that many unpleasant or undesirable conditions once thought just part of ordinary life can now be medically treated (getting old, pattern baldness), and (3) that there are new drugs or devices in the pipeline that will dramatically improve our lives. Donald L. Bartlett and James B. Steele, summarizing the advertisements and health warnings from a variety of sources, found that if we add up all the warning alarms about hypertension, osteoporosis, incontinence, herpes, irritable bowl syndrome, sleep disorders, restless leg syndrome, latent tuberculosis infection, atrial fibrillation, liver disease . . . and another dozen or so conditions, we would have to conclude that "there are more than 1.5 billion sick people in the United States—or five times the population. . . . Are Americans really that sick? Of course not. . . . it's in the interest of a market-driven medical system to make you think you are sick, or soon will be, or to worry you over the possibility."[11] If that statement seems overly cynical, it may well be that a parallel interpretation, a bit softer, might be that medical progress steadily raises the standards of what counts as good and bad health and that the bad always outweighs the good: doing better and feeling worse.

The sociologist Peter Conrad, a pioneer analyst of medicalization, has defined it as a "process by which nonmedical problems become defined and treated as medical problems, usually in terms of illness and disorders."[12] He notes that when he first became interested in the issue in the 1970s there was "no mention of now common maladies such as attention-deficit/hyperactivity disorder (ADHD), fetal alcohol syndrome, premenstrual syndrome (PMS), and sudden infant death syndrome (SIDS), [nor were] obesity or alcoholism widely viewed in the medical profession as a disease."[13]

The most important developments he has observed since then are the expansion of the category of life problems now designated as diseases, and the dominant role of industry in broadening the category and then aggressively marketing a treatment for them (usually a drug). The FDA approved the drug Paxil in 1996 for the treatment of depression, but its manufacturer (now called GlaxoSmithKline), asked the FDA for permission extend its use into the "anxiety market." At first that encompassed panic disorder and obsessive compulsive disorder and then moved on to include social anxiety disorder (SAD) and generalized anxiety disorder (GAD), and finally the anxiety market contributed to "the medicalization" of emotions such as worry and shyness. The drug eventually ran into some safety problems but not before it helped to establish a whole range of new medical pathologies.

Conrad wisely does not pretend to claim that these are not "medical" conditions, but only that it was clever marketing (with some professional blessing) that led to the deployment of therapies for these conditions. Moreover, I would add, it is possible to say that, for instance, aging is not a disease but a normal and natural part of life and yet at the same time target all of the unpleasant features of aging as is if they are. One can thus say that any and all features of our life that we find distasteful are potential targets for medical intervention and treatment. The medical industry, Conrad shows, has now replaced the medical profession and various other groups and social movements as the prime mover: "the engines of medicalization have proliferated and are now driven more by commercial and market interests than by professional claims-makers."[14]

THE FAILURE OF REFORM EFFORTS

The charges and complaints against the medical industry have done little good. There have been some successful efforts to keep drug company representatives away from medical students, to limit visits to hospitals and doctor's offices by "detail" people (pharmaceutical company salespeople), to set limits on free meals and other perks for physicians, to stop publications on research that have obvious conflict-of-interest problems, and to set some industry guidelines on marketing behavior. They are helpful, but not enough.

There are a variety of reasons for the general failure to effect large scale reforms. There is the obvious fact that many legislators receive campaign contributions, that the industry does only what other industries do (even if more so), and that most of its dubious practices are not illegal, however offensive they may seem (and thus there is little effective leverage against them). An industry that wraps itself in the dual royal mantles of market freedom and life-saving products has everything going for it. To say, moreover, that it is an industry which, in its aggressive marketing and political efforts, is harmful is not to say that its products are; and that distinction is the drug industry's ace in the hole, for which so much is forgiven.

The biotechnology and medical device industries have not been the target of such concerted criticism, perhaps because they are a bit more removed from direct interaction with the public and have also avoided some of the more egregious marketing practices of the drug industry (although they are formidable lobbyists). But the aggressiveness of device companies in selling their products (e.g., imaging devices) and their ability to win the business of physicians and hospitals has not gone unnoticed (see chapter 3). Their products are generally expensive, particularly those designed to provide care for the most critically ill, itself the most expensive portion of the patient population. Hospital ICUs are a veritable showcase for its products.

The biotechnology industry, a relative newcomer hardly more than 30 years old, has been notable for a number of special features. It took a long time to get off the ground, and its companies absorbed large amounts of money from venture capitalists over many years before turning a profit. These companies were also in the vanguard of luring academic scientists into industry, many of whom themselves became entrepreneurs, creating their own start-up companies. These scientists thus broke from a long tradition in medicine and biology of looking down their noses at the for-profit sector and at making large amounts of money. While the pharmaceutical industry always had academic researchers and advisors, the excitement of biotechnology, a new scientific frontier, and the emerging spirit of the Reagan years in 1980s that lionized entrepreneurs and the accumulation of wealth gave the field an entirely different flavor. Its possibilities excited Wall Street and university scientists alike, and many universities began to open offices to take part in the projected largesse. The market had come to the academy, perhaps not quite rivaling big time sports and the salaries of coaches that exceeded those of college presidents, but it was trying.

The biotechnology industry has run into what seems to me a special problem, not unknown in the other industries by any means, but greatly intensified, that of very expensive products. Although it may have created some inexpensive products, I have not heard of them. Instead, we have begun hearing of a rising number of drugs whose costs can run into tens of thousands of dollars. Genentech's drug Avastin, for the treatment of colorectal and lung cancer, costs close to $50,000 for a 10-month course of treatment. The Celgene Company has a drug for multiple myeloma that costs $67,000 for its use. Another Genentech product, Lucentis, provides treatment for macular degeneration for a price of $48,000 for 2 years. Genentech rationalized its high price for Avastin on the grounds that "life is priceless," a novel ethical argument that brought cat calls, as if that made it economically justifiable.[15]

Jerry Avorn of the Harvard Medical School has pointed out that many of the expensive genetic-based biotechnologies were developed in part by the federal government but with no payback to it for doing so, and no inclination on the part of the industry to do so.[16] Is that not what "big government" is all about, at least when it wants to support industry, but a different story when it comes to price control? To rub it in a bit, the industry has resisted the development of biotechnology generics, which means the companies have a virtual monopoly on their own products and can market them at a high price without fear of competition.[17] Joseph Newhouse, after reviewing and rejecting a variety of possible ways to set drug prices, opts instead for Congress to allow costs to be considered in coverage decisions.[18] He surely knows the long history of failures to move Congress in that direction, but it is such a commonsensical approach that its logic can hardly be denied.

James C. Mullen, CEO of Biogen Idec and, in 2007, chairman of BIO, said in a speech to some founders of younger and smaller companies that "You haven't done anything wrong—your products don't cost too much. . . . You are the underdogs in a David and Goliath story . . . America loves this story." He is right about the love part, but not necessarily the rest. But that love, especially when combined with the tactic of keeping critics sullen but not mutinous, is hard to beat.

PHYSICIANS AND MONEY

The complex relationship between physicians and industry goes well beyond their being prime targets for industry marketing. All of us are subject to advertising of one kind or another, and we are, we usually believe, smart enough to know when to listen and when to turn off. Physicians have long said that they are not affected by advertisements, detail men, free meals, and occasional junkets. I suspect all of us think we are much too savvy to be suckered in by such pressures, and maybe that is often true. Nonetheless, it is evident that the medical industries think otherwise. Why would they keep doing it if it were a waste of money? They have studied us more rigorously than we have studied them, and that same confident savvy we think we have might be inferior to their study of us, and probably is. A charming detail man, pushing a new drug and generously handing out samples, may be quite persuasive to harassed and busy doctors, much too busy to check out the sales pitch in medical journals. He knows the pressure his physician target is under and well understands that a good personal pitch is usually more effective than a journal analysis, which he can be reasonably confident the doctor has not, and probably will not, read.

That problem can be dealt with, if not entirely, and steps are underway to do so. More complex are some other variables. The most basic is trying to determine the extent to which physicians have been influenced by an affluence-driven culture; that is, are they so in tune with our society that they have a view of money and economic status that has been shaped, not by the history and traditions of medicine, but by the values of the society in which they are imbedded and about which they may be no less unaware of its influence than the rest of us? The other question, at a very different level, is the extent to which organized medicine—by which I mean medical associations and societies, which have more political power than individual physicians—have a compromised relationship with industry.

I will open this analysis with my own observations of, and reading about, physicians. I offer some of this as anecdotal evidence, the only kind available. How, I have long asked myself, do doctors think about money? I observe four groups. First, physicians whose main goal it is to serve patients well, and to do so without a great concern for money. They can be found in health care organizations whose physicians are salaried, in the military and Veterans Administration, and heavily in the fields of pediatrics, internal medicine, geriatrics, rehabilitation, and family practice. They are, in short, in medical fields and organizations where there are built-in limits on income and comparatively few economic incentives or possibilities to make a great deal of money.

Second, there are those who do seek a good living, far better than average, and have a strong sense of entitlement: I worked hard to get where I am, ran up large education debts, and believe there is no incompatibility between a good, very good, living and good patient care. This is the territory of cardiac and thoracic surgery, oncology, radiology, dermatology, and gastrointestinal medicine. This is the group for whom fee-for-service medicine, being paid one procedure at a time, is most lucrative.

Third, there are those who are outright entrepreneurs, opening their own clinics or specialty hospitals and who, in every way, work to maximize their income. They may continue treating individual patients, but many become full-time managers.

Fourth, although the borderlines are fluid, cutting across each of the categories above, are those who work through existing general and medical specialty groups to improve the working conditions and income of physicians in those groups, but with some seemingly more oriented to the income side.

Worries about the commercialization of medicine have been around for many years, but they have increased of late. There have always been young people who went into medicine as a good route to a good income or those who, once in it, began to see financial possibilities that they earlier had not imagined. I believe a change began to emerge by the 1960s. Medicine had by then become part of a health care system that was commanding huge portions of the national income, and it was evident that there was money to be made. The Medicare program was itself a great stimulus to increased physician incomes, particularly because it was heavily oriented to fee-for-service remuneration. Once making money became more acceptable in the wider society, it became more acceptable in medicine as well; and there was more money than ever to be made. An earlier stigma had all but vanished.

The 1980s, the Reagan years, were important as an accelerant, a time when the making of money was celebrated and taken as the best sign of professional success, and when market thinking began to rush like a flood into almost every realm of American life. Rapid progress in medical technology, and its effective selling by industry, fit very nicely into the broader embrace of money, offering more and more ways of making more of it, particularly for medical specialists. The industry itself became an important employer of physicians, many of whom have risen high in managerial positions with salaries commensurate with those of other major industries. Physician CEOs salaries that are well over a $1 million a year are growing number. The distinguished Editor Emeritus of the *New England Journal of Medicine*, Dr. Arnold S. Relman, spent much of his career speaking out against the commercialization of medicine, not just against industry, but many of his colleagues as well. He considers "the transformation of the U.S. health care system from a professional service for the sick and injured into one of the country's largest industries to be the most important socioeconomic change in the last half century of health care in our country."[19] The medical historian Rosemary A. Stevens has examined in useful detail the "gulf between a health care 'industry' and 'social' medicine."[20]

Three examples of the force of money stand out: physician-owned medical specialty hospitals, the increase of technological procedures performed by physicians, and growing disparities in different medical specialties.

Physician-Owned Specialty Hospitals

Physician-owned specialty hospitals are a good example of the problems caused by entrepreneurial physicians. In 1972, the federal government began to impose a number of laws and regulations aiming to prohibit physicians from referring their Medicare and Medicaid patients to free-standing facilities in which a physician or family member has an investment interest.[21] There were a few exceptions, most notably what became known as the "whole-hospital exception," which encompassed specialty hospitals, most notably cardiac, orthopedic, surgical, and gynecological facilities. That exception did not sit well with general hospitals: exactly the same range of services were among the most profitable for them. A combination of dissatisfaction among physicians about the way hospitals treated them and an outright profit motive were behind the development of the specialty hospitals. By 2003, there were 100 such hospitals nationally, with another 26 under development.

One important result of this development was almost open warfare between general and specialty hospitals. "We are," a Miami hospital executive wrote, "in competition with our own medical staff."[22] The physicians may compete by owning or working for specialty hospitals or ambulatory surgical and ambulatory centers. Doctors, some reports contend, once had loyalty to a hospital, but now treat their office as the center of their professional activity. Not only may the loyalty to a specific hospital be diminishing but also an important source of hospital income as well in the growing difficulty in getting specialist physicians to provide emergency room service. "A major source of wasted spending," one study found, "lies in unwarranted intensity of hospital and physician services, particularly for patients in the last month of life. . . . physicians have renewed a 'medical arms race' that is driving up costs even faster, sometimes as collaborators but increasingly as competitors."[23]

Jeff Goldsmith, President of Health Futures, paints an even darker picture. "A new and deeply exploitative model of medical practice," he writes, "is emerging in some physician communities, particularly in the Sun Belt . . . 'lecture fees,' free travel and other perks from drug companies to promote new drugs to physician colleagues, 'consulting fees' from device manufacturers to use their products exclusively . . . and 'stipends' from hospitals for critical care coverage that physicians used to provide voluntarily."[24] Noting various efforts to combat this situation, Goldsmith and Berenson would eliminate Medicare "reimbursement windfalls" for services, particularly cardiac care, as well as providing possible tax benefits for physicians proportionate to their community services. A study of physician self-referrals to services they had a financial stake in, although prohibited by federal law in the early 1990s, revealed that a variety of ways were devised to evade it, particularly with advanced imaging procedures.[25] I have focused here on specialty hospitals. The full store would include diagnostic imaging centers, ambulatory surgery centers, and MRI units in physician offices.

TRENDS IN PHYSICIAN PROCEDURES

In 1992, Medicare initiated a resource-based relative value scale, basing its payments on the relative units of value (RUVs) assigned to physician services. It was based on a combination of the volume of physician work, practice expenses, and professional liability insurance.[26] It was introduced in response to the widespread complaints that physicians were underpaid for evaluation and management services and, for those who performed procedures, overpaid; and there was a fear that this imbalance was leading toward a shortage of primary care physicians. The RUV plan has not worked out as hoped. Between 1992 and 2002, the volume of physician's work per beneficiary grew by 50% and the total RUVs per Medicare beneficiary by 50%.

The quantity and mix of services were the main sources of growth: physicians were doing more things for patients and doing them more intensively. Cardiology and gastroenterology accounted for the greatest growth of physicians work.[27] While the quantity of evaluation and management services increased by 18% between 1992–2002, the quantity of imaging services rose by 70% and nonmajor procedures by 21%. The net result has been that payments to physicians for management and evaluation have remained static, while those for procedures have sharply increased. Joseph P. Newhouse has predicted that economic pressures on Medicare will keep spending on physician services modest, but that will not necessarily happen with procedures because of the fee-for-service policy that provides incentives to use them.[28] Some of the increase in procedures has come from an increase in their scope, but most has come from just doing more of what pays best. That is an old story, ever refreshed with new or updated technologies and one surely intensified by industry success by advertising in enlarging the pool of the worried well.

PRIMARY CARE MEDICINE

In the next chapter, I argue that the royal road to lower health care costs is to push as much care as possible to the lowest possible level of basic care. The role of primary care is critical to doing this. Save for emergency hospital care, it is to primary care physicians that most patients go when worried about their health, either because of specific symptoms or more general health anxieties. At some point in our life, sooner or later, we will all have to go to them. But in American health care, it is a discipline in retreat, beset by decreasing numbers, patient difficulty of gaining access, competition from medical subspecialties, and a weak financial position in relation to them.

A long-standing ideal of medical care is that of a "sustained relationship between patients and the clinicians who care for them."[29] In 1976, when the idea of primary care was first being formalized, 88% of adults reported having a "regular source" of care, most of them a particular physician or a facility with several physicians to play that role.[30] Central to the primary care ideal is that of a "whole person" orientation, which combines a long-term commitment with a holistic perspective on the health of a patient in the context of that patient's life. In the eyes of patients, that orientation is now not always present. Based on some patient surveys, only about one-third of them consider their physician's knowledge of them to be excellent or good—and that despite "considerable continuity" in their relationship with a physician.[31] Most alarmingly, two studies of Medicare beneficiaries covering the periods 1996–1999 and 1998–2000 found "substantial decline in financial access to care, visit-based continuity, and integration of care."[32] That decline suggests, in the words of Safran that "we are far from the ideal of primary care that is whole-person oriented, and we appear to be losing ground."[33]

There are some obvious reasons why this is happening. The internal pressures on primary care physicians are enormous. They range from mastering a basic knowledge of medical problems across a wide range of subdisciplines, always generating new information, the care of patients with complicated long-term chronic and degenerative diseases, and the pressure of a practice financially determined by the quantity of their services and not necessarily by its quality.[34]

That last feature, characteristic of fee-for-service medicine, is little more than piece work. Time spent performing a diagnostic, surgical, or imaging procedure can pay three times as much as dealing with chronic conditions or simply talking with patients to better understand their needs. Between 1995 and 2004, the median income for primary care physicians increased by 21.4% compared with 37.5% for specialists. It is hardly surprising that, with financial prospects of that kind, there is a decline in medical students going into the primary care field. Between 1997 and 2005, the number of medical students going into family practice residencies decreased by 50%. The more technology a doctor can wield, and the more expensive the technology, the greater that physician's income.

As Thomas Bodenheimer notes, there is another kind of fallout as well: "many nurse practitioners and physicians who could join the primary care workforce are instead going to work in wealthier specialty practices. Primary care practices in the United States now depend on luring physicians away from other countries."[35] The shift from primary to subspecialty care is a shift from less expensive, technology-light, care to more expensive technology-heavy care. "A strong primary care infrastructure," Dr. Beverly Woo has written, "is associated with better health outcomes, lower costs, and a more equitable health care system," a point underlined by European health care, with a much higher ratio of primary-to-specialist physicians.[36] The ratio of primary-to-specialists in the United States is about 30:70 versus 60:40 in the United Kingdom and 50:50 in most other countries.

But, Woo notes, a decreasing job satisfaction, increasing medical school debts, and growing salary disparities "could together create a strong sense that becoming a primary care physician may be a fool's errand."[37] The notion, moreover, that physician specialists, particularly in anesthesiology and obstetric/gynecology, are being driven from the field because of high malpractice insurance costs (far less a problem with primary care physicians) has little empirical evidence to support it.[38] The financial incentives for specialty practices remain powerful and those for primary care weak. A shortage of 25,000–40,000 primary care practices has been projected.[39]

MEDICINE, MONEY, AND MORALS

There are for me two leading puzzles in trying to understand and reform the medical industry and medical professionalism. One of them is the most obvious: if we grant, as I will, that the very market practices espoused by the medical industry that are the most worthy of condemnation are themselves closely related to the medical benefits of its research and technological innovations, how might these be disentangled—if that is even possible? The other conundrum is that if the practice of medicine is closely related to a medical industry that supplies it with many of the technological tools needed to practice good medicine, then how can medicine as a profession retain its traditional core value of patient welfare above all else? Can those tools be used at arm's length from the industry that produces them? In theory, yes, in practice it is difficult. The mix of money, market realities, and medicine creates the difficulty.

THE MARKET AND THE MEDICAL INDUSTRY

In chapters 3 and 4 I discussed the long-standing debate about whether the provision of health care is an appropriate place for a full-scale deployment of market values and practices. That is an important debate, but there is an analogous one we should be having. Is the market the best instrument for pursuing the improvement of health and the reduction of illness? That is a different question from asking if market practices can deliver fair and efficient health care at an affordable price. We might, in short, hold that the market and its characteristic practices are poorly adaptable to the provision of care, but suitable for the development and dissemination of the technological means necessary for that provision. If that latter possibility is plausible, then one can ask: can a market-driven industry provide its goods, services, and technologies in a way that does not do harm to the health care system which makes use of them, and that can control its costs. Not easily.

Historically, there has always been a private market to provide medical instruments, drugs, and devices. For the most part it was made up of modest enterprises, and at times producing treatments of little value, and sometimes even harmful, for a patient's health. The medical industry as we know it today can best be traced to the emergence of the German pharmaceutical industry during the last half of the nineteenth century. It was an industry that did good research, produced (for the time) good drugs, and pioneered many marketing techniques that served as a model for later industries. But while the German drug companies skillfully worked with universities and government, they were private enterprises; and so they remained, as did almost all other medical industries. On occasion in various countries government took on the role of developing and producing medical products; this often occurred during wartime or in the context of the need, say, for vaccines against influenza and other potential epidemics.

The great shift, from relatively small industries of little national economic importance to large ones of great importance, came in the aftermath of World War II. The NIH in the United States emerged as a powerful source of basic biomedical research with the understanding that the results of that research would be used by industry to develop its clinical applications. There would be no quid for quo. Industry was free to use the NIH research largesse to generate its products without recompense to the government. American taxpayers are now paying the bill for the basic research. And although industry was of course happy to accept that government benefit, it was otherwise opposed to government intervention and regulation (which it often got, like it or not) but was most successful, as we have seen, in opposing price controls and resisting economic assessments of technology.

Arrangements of that kind introduced into American health care a fundamental clash of values. The medical industry wanted, and still wants, to be treated like any other industry, free to sell its products to whomever will buy them, free to advertise and merchandise them like any other industry, and free to lobby to promote its self-interest the way every other industry does. But unlike most other industries, it has proclaimed better health, not profit, as its real goal. Everyone knows that is not quite the full story. Because its products are crucial for health and generally work well toward that end, the industry has been more or less allowed to retain the values of the market, often in its most raw form, while proclaiming its commitment to the altruistic values of traditional medicine.

But those values are in conflict in a harmful way. The fact that we all benefit from its pursuit of profits does not justify what that pursuit does to American health care, which is to help drive up health care costs to a dangerous level, which then works to harm the very health it proclaims to serve. I see no way out of this conflict other than to begin classifying medical industries much as we do some public utilities, that is, as private companies that perform a public good. The latter are lauded for their public benefit but regulated with an eye to making certain that their quest for profits does not harm their important public role. The Dutch relationship between insurance companies and the government embodies that model.

INDUSTRY AND THE MEDICAL PROFESSION

The relationship between the medical profession and industry is symbiotic: each needs the other. Physicians need industry to provide the technologies and treatments to pursue their profession. Industry needs physicians as the necessary pathway to patients. Even with direct-to-consumer advertising there is, with prescription drugs, the necessary rule that one must "consult one's physician." There is thus no easy way for either industry or the profession to avoid each other, or to avoid an intimate relationship. Yet if they are in a relationship that can be exceedingly beneficial to both, they are also in a relationship that can be more harmful to the profession of medicine than to the medical industry. I doubt that industry could, by itself, seduce physicians down the commercialization trail. But in an American culture that makes much of making money, offers many things to spend it on, and has persuaded more and more physicians over the years that there is nothing wrong with doing good and doing well, medicine and commerce become congenial partners.

The ideal solution is that of salaried physicians or physicians working in capitated practices, able to make a decent living without having to multiply profitable technological procedures. But the deepest American tradition has been fee-for-service medicine, not only profitable but drawing upon the enduring vision of a medical practice that focuses on the unique characteristics of doctor–patient relationship. That relationship draws upon the belief that all patients are different, and that compensation for treating them should have differential payments.

But there is one point about which there is considerable agreement: the worst possible system to control costs is a fee-for-service payment system embedded in third-party payments—the standard model for most health insurance plans and policies. Patients do not have to worry about the cost of their treatment, from which they are sheltered, and doctors benefit from payment policies rewarding technological procedures, not the kind of time and effort it takes to oversee and coordinate long-term chronic illness, which is just the kind of illness almost surely to be the dominant feature of the care of the retired baby boomers in the near future.

Although future compensatory arrangements will surely need to be changed, a basic question is this: can the traditional ethic of medicine, patient centered and altruistic, survive in a market-dominated, money-loving society? That latter combination is predicated on a profit-oriented industry abetted by a medical profession eager to take every advantage of the good money that a sophisticated physician can make if he has a sharp eye for economic opportunities and few hesitations about taking advantage of them. Why not? Why should doctors be different, at least in the way they think about money and the good life, than everyone else who makes socially valuable contributions?

Arnold S. Relman has, in an "open letter" to his medical colleagues, proposed the creation of multispecialty prepaid group practices, and payment of physicians with salaries rather than fee-for-service remuneration.[40] "Rejecting any self-serving financial connections with clinical facilities outside your own group practice or group . . . You should return to the old precept that 'a practicing physician's professional income should be derived entirely from direct services or from the supervision of such services.' "[41] Dr. Relman's recommendations to his colleagues seem to me eminently sensible. Whether they can take hold is not clear; they certainly would not be easy to implement.

Is it possible to transform a profession that, unwittingly or not, has become at least in part the hand-maiden of the medical industry? I am not certain about whether that will happen, or even whether it could happen, but I am certain it must happen. I do not expect the medical industry (to understate the probabilities) to take a lead in such a transformation; nor, unhappily, do I expect all of the mainline medical professional (and thus advocacy) groups to join a common effort to clean up the Augean stables of a commercialized medicine. As long as the current system is in place, technology has a free ride with medicine and commerce living together in a comfortable cohabitation relationship.

CHAPTER 6

✺

"MEDICAL NECESSITY"

AN ALL-BUT-USELESS CONCEPT

The United States, it is often said, has no real health care system, at least if that means a centrally organized system with an integrated set of institutions and practices.

As a general characterization, that statement is true enough. But our hybrid arrangements, mixing private and public values and organizing principles, do have a deep-seated set of cultural values, reflecting a long history of tension and struggle. The principal values are choice and individualism, but with an important qualification, that of the necessity of government to support care for the poor and the elderly. But even the latter has in practice an embedded individualistic bias, effectively limiting the power of government to intervene in doctor–patient relationships or to judge the value and validity of personal patient decisions, which I will call patient self-definition decisions.

That bias, I will argue, has made it difficult to give anything more than an amorphous meaning to critical legal and policy concepts such as "medical necessity" or "reasonable and necessary" (the language of Medicare legislation), thus making it almost impossible to come to grips with technology costs. That failure, in turn, reflects the long-standing unwillingness in this country—most pronounced in the failure of Congress to allow cost as a consideration in Medicare benefit coverage decisions—to take cost into serious account in our health policy. To do that would mean saying "no" to medical wants and desires, and some real needs as well. To move in that direction would require a recognition of the social and collective nature of health care and its provision and the urgent need to find ways to set limits. "Medical necessity" and "reasonable and necessary" are wholly oriented to individual patient welfare, not the common good of the health care system. That individualist orientation, when joined as it is with a cultural commitment to unlimited technological innovation, simply makes it impossible in practice to control costs, but also in principle rules it out.

My central contention, underlying this chapter and the next, is that we will be unable to deal effectively with the rising cost of medical technology unless we significantly change our view of health care. We need to move from what I call an infinity model—unlimited medical progress and technological innovation—to a finite model, one that understands the necessity to shape health care goals that are affordable, accessible, and sustainable. How should we understand the concept of medical necessity? It is widely used as a standard for determining what treatments patients should receive, and what technologies should be covered by private health insurance or government programs. But it is an open-end standard that neither in principle nor in practice can cope with new and ever-changing technologies.

Our health care reformers are now trying to do the impossible: to find a way to manage a health care system that is saturated with the elixir of technology, where there is no such thing as enough, and to find managerial and organizational ways to make that addiction affordable and accessible. That cannot be done. Instead, we need to envision a finite model and work from there to develop organizational means of implementing it. Our first and perhaps most fundamental challenge is to understand the way the value of individual self-definition makes the larger task of system reform all but impossible but also why that value cannot be changed without a simultaneous organizational change.

Technology often gives us what we desire—better health, and hence health itself has become equated with technology, a necessary if not sufficient condition for health. Of course there are alternatives to technology as a route to health. There is prevention, and there is also improvement of socioeconomic conditions. But for most people, the burning question is: what will be done to me and for me when I might become sick, or when I do become sick? That is where technology comes in. But what happens as that relationship becomes increasingly unaffordable, indeed unsustainable economically? We have some choices. We can try to change our personal values, tutoring ourselves to want something different in the name of health, using economic necessity as an impetus. Or we can try to change the health care system to one that has different values. Or we can aim for some mixture of the two. It is that last possibility I want to explore in this chapter and the next, if only because it is unimaginable that we could hope to devise a different kind of health care system, undergirded by different values, without changing our current individual values. Without such a change, there would be a destructive dissonance as the two move in opposing directions.

There are four features of the technology dynamic that must be reexamined at both the personal and the public policy level. One of them is the individual desire for constant progress, a craving for the latest and the best technology has to offer—a desire that seems insatiable. The second is that of the health policy level, where research is funded, insurance coverage is provided (public and private), and resources allocated. The third is the professional level, which bears on the values, education, and acculturation of physicians and other health care workers. The fourth is that of the commercial health care industry, ranging from insurance providers to managers of for-profit facilities all the way through the various industries that develop and sell medical technologies.

None of those issues can meaningfully be addressed without some picture in our minds of what values a health care system should embody. What are the individual and social goals it seeks? What is it meant to contribute to our human condition, one marked by illness, aging, and death, all fearful prospects? A common picture often invoked is a list of ideal features of a health care system, for instance that it should be accessible, equitable, universal, and economically sustainable. These might aptly be called the social and economic values that ought to underlie health care. They are surely important values, and I have invoked them myself earlier in this book. But there are still deeper strata that are important. One of them is that of the moral and political principles meant to establish a person's claim to health care and the obligation of others to provide it. Here the most common language and concepts have been justice and equity, empathy, human rights, and solidarity (most common in Europe), and they have been helpful.

DEFINING A FINITE MODEL OF HEALTH CARE

The other stratum, and the one I take to be primary, consists of a view of human nature and life and of the place that the quest for health should have in it. The most prevalent view is one I have called the "infinity model" of health care.[1] By that I mean an open-ended view of medical progress and technological innovation, one that has no finite goals, no inherent limits to aspirations for better health, and no shared notion of the meaning of such common terms as "good health," the "quality of life," and "medical necessity."

In one sense, that lack of shared meaning bespeaks a culture of medical relativism and political pluralism; those are the values that individualistic, free societies generate, although more intensively in America than in other developed countries. Even more, it reflects a utopian vision of science and its possibilities. There is no disease that cannot be cured, no length of life that cannot be aspired to, no human enhancement that is beyond the realm of scientific possibility, and no biologically based mental or physical suffering that cannot be overcome. One consequence of this view is not simply its emotional power in pushing us continually forward—for who wants to get sick, to suffer, to die?—but no less the grip this aspirational model has on our conscience: it would be profoundly wrong, many argue, not to pursue the unlimited possibilities to improve health, combat aging, and to carry out a war against death.[2]

Yet that infinity model is increasingly unaffordable—nearing the limits of economic plausibility—and with a destructive distortion of our other important national needs. To make the doctor's office and health care the center of American life would not be a good outcome. The assorted managerial efforts to control costs, pointed out in previous chapters, are not working in the United States and are barely working even in those countries that use the strongest available means. Those realities should alert us to the inherent difficulties of trying to finance an infinity model of health care with finite funds.

We need a new and different model, one that is limited in aspiration and thus economically more plausible but at the same time still responsive to our need for good health. Here are my ingredients for such a model. At its core is an acceptance of the reality of death and aging, which we can aim to ameliorate, not conquer. I start with the assumption, earlier uncontroversial but now more contentious, that we are biologically finite creatures, born to live but eventually to die, and whose lives as a whole should be valued more for what is done with them than for how long they last.

The aim of health care should be, within a finite life span, to help us to have a good chance to progress from being young to being old—but not to go from being old to being indefinitely older; to relieve us of our most burdensome physical and mental suffering—but not always fully or perfectly; to rehabilitate us as best it can if we are disabled—but to understand that some of us will live our lives with chronic illnesses and disabilities; and to help us achieve as pain-free and peaceful death as is possible—but knowing that goal will not always be possible. Medicine ought not to seek an indefinite extension of life, or aim to enhance our nature beyond the ordinary standards of good health, or search out medical ways of excessively fighting our decline and frailties, many of which are now and always will be unavoidable. Just as death ought not to be taken as the ultimate enemy of human life, health should not be taken as the ultimate good.

As this chapter and the next move along, I spell out more details of the finite model, and particularly what it might entail in the way we live our lives and manage our institutions, including a health care system that deploys technology as its primary means of pursuing health. I begin with two general and fundamental premises, in deep tension with each other. One of them was well articulated by the great biologist Rene Dubos. In his book *The Mirage of Health*, Dubos wrote that "complete and lasting freedom from disease is but a dream remembered from imaginings of a Garden of Eden."[3] It is not an accident that we are subject to disease. It is an inherent biological feature of human life, as much a part of that life as the good health we sporadically achieve. Decline and decay, growth and flourishing, are parts of our human nature.

My other premise is an astute observation by the political scientist Michael Walzer. "What has happened in the modern world," he wrote, "is simply that disease itself, even when it is endemic rather than epidemic, has come to be seen as a plague. And since the plague can be dealt with, it *must* be dealt with. People will not endure what they no longer believe they have to endure."[4]

In those two premises we can see the perfect psychological and social dilemma. We can never entirely conquer disease and mortality, which always bring us down in the end. Nor can we stop trying. The possibility of the first would require fashioning ourselves into a different kind of organic creature, as yet undiscovered; but we can do something, maybe very much, to relieve our situation, and we feel compelled to try. How do we balance these two powerful cross currents in light of the cost problem and do so with each of the four dimensions noted above: the personal, the policy, the professional, and the commercial?

SHAPING OUR PERSONAL HEALTH CARE VALUES

Our times are rife with the notion of a consumer-directed medicine. It aims to put greater choice into our individual hands, facilitated by a wide range of competitive providers to give us the kind of care we want. Oddly missing is any serious discussion about what kind of care we *should* want. How should I think about my health, and what kind of priority should it have in my life? I am not, however, thinking about two kinds of discussions that seem to respond to questions of that kind: that of the choices we should be able to make in our end-of-life care, or in selecting a doctor or hospital or in choosing specialized care.

Those values, turning on our right to make certain choices, are important but are of second order. They do not bear on the specific content or substance of our choices but, rather, on the *kind* of options that should be available to us. In much of the political debate about choices, it is assumed that, once we have choice, the substance of that choice is a matter of personal decision. It is a choice that no one but ourselves should be free to make, and the standards for doing so are our own, whether these standards seem wise or good in the eyes of others. I will be allowed to choose an all-but-useless and painful round of chemotherapy should I so decide, or decline a useful and painless round also should I so choose. Or I might be an independent consultant with three young children and a nonworking wife, but without employer-provided health insurance; if I choose, I will be allowed to buy a cheap, barely adequate family policy even if I have foolishly decided to spend my money instead to pay for an expensive family boat or swimming pool; or to buy no policy at all. Those are the kinds of choice celebrated in America, embraced by liberals as an expression of human freedom and by conservatives as the moral basis of a market economy. We will have differing opinions on the wisdom or prudence of the choices made by others, but rarely do we disagree on their right to make them.

The terrible difficulty with that kind of legal and moral stance is twofold. Such a position makes it exceedingly hard to establish health care policies meant to satisfy everyone (of which more later). It no less means that we get practically no help from our neighbor or our society about what might best count as a good or bad choice, a prudent or unwise choice, or a choice that is beneficial only to ourselves over against one that might be more beneficial to our community. We act as if freedom and pluralism, with some help from the market, rule out that kind of public discourse.

What Ought We Choose When We Are Free to Choose?

I realize that many Americans cherish this country precisely because it offers the kind of pluralism, and even moral relativism, that allows us to live our lives as we choose. Such a society is surely preferable to more autocratic, authoritarian regimes, even if it generates many civil, moral, and legal problems. But moral pluralism is of little help to us in deciding how personally to live and how to die and, particularly, how to live and die in the company of contemporary health care.

We need to have some help with first-order questions of that kind. It is good that our hospitals and doctors will give us some choice about how we die. But do not expect them to answer the following questions. Once I have a choice, when *ought* I want to die? What do I owe others as part of that decision? How much physical pain *ought* I be willing to bear in order to spare my family psychological pain? Do I owe it to my family to undergo as many diagnostic procedures as possible in order to preserve my life, even if the odds are low that some or many will find anything pathological?

Here are some of my answers. I *ought* to want to die when—overcome by illness—I have lived a reasonably full life, when I have discharged my main obligations to my family and friends, when my death would seem neither premature nor tragic to others. I would also want to die in a way that presented the least possible burden to my family, and yet accept the possibility that, against my will, I could well be a burden. In that case I would expect my family to accept that burden, just as I would be prepared to bear the burden of their dying. I should also be willing to put up with some physical pain as long as I could possibly bear it, that is, to the point where it begins to be wholly absorbing my attention and destroying my personhood.

I believe I have an obligation at our moment in history, and at my stage of life (age 79), to make use of as little expensive technology as possible, using only that technology that will do me significant good and not just add a few more months of life. I therefore resist heavy diagnostic screening to turn up asymptomatic problems, and no less resist follow-up treatment of the low-probability "better safe than sorry" variety.

DEATH AND MEDICAL TECHNOLOGY

Human beings have a characteristic and biologically long-lasting life cycle, one that we will all go through if we do not die a premature death. Simply put, we are born, become children, adolescents, and then adults, and finally become old. For centuries that course has been depicted as one of advancing up a ladder, with mature adulthood as the top point, then down the ladder to death. Our life span is much longer now than earlier, some 78 years on average in the United States, but the ladder is still much the same shape, although descent from it tapers off more slowly now in old age.

Death, however, has become an unforeseen puzzle for contemporary medicine. For centuries medicine could do little about death, limited to some diagnostic skills and simple forms of care. By the end of the nine-teenth century, however, cures were becoming possible, and their pace increased dramatically in the twentieth century. During that same time frame, life expectancies increased 40 years or so from a combination of medical progress and improved public health and socioeconomic devel-opments. While it is hard to pin down a specific date, I believe that some-where in the 1960s and early 1970s two changes took place with a third to follow in the 1990s that began to alter the way medicine and the public looked at death.[5]

One of these changes was a rhetorical escalation in the struggle against death and a rapid increase in the research budget of the NIH directed particularly against the leading lethal conditions of cancer and heart disease, and death was turned into the main enemy not just of health but, it came to seem, of human life itself. Richard Nixon's declara-tion of "war" against cancer in 1970 stands as a symbol of that change in intensity. It was during that era also that I first heard the phrase "research imperative," meant to convey the idea that there was now a moral obligation to fight death and disease and that the scientific means were at hand to do so.[6] Medical technology was the weapon of choice for that war, pushed along by the research imperative: we can do it, and we ought to do it.

The second change in the 1960s and 1970s was the increasingly blurred line between living and dying, an important reason for the eruption of interest in that era to end-of-life care. The growing capacity of medical technology to extend life always a bit longer even with the sickest patients created ethical problems in the termination of care. The move from a heart–lung definition of death to that of a whole brain definition nicely symbolizes that development. Heart–lung machines could by then sustain respiration and blood circulation for long periods of time in the absence of brain activity, thus requiring a new definition to adapt to the technological development. More generally, constant advances in medical technology were able to extend life longer and longer, often making it hard to know when a physician should stop treatment. An important medical anthropology study by Barbara Koenig and a colleague of physicians caring for the dying found that a patient is not even defined as dying until the clinician determines "that there are no more [technological] interventions that will improve the patient's condition."[7]

The Cure of Utopianism

Death is then not something that only happens to bodies from biological causes; it no less comes from the absence of technologies to stop it. Perhaps this phenomenon is best seen in cancer treatment, where the attraction of "one more round" of chemotherapy, based on the slimmest of hopes, is often undertaken: the patient will not die unless that treatment fails. The shift in thinking is subtle but momentous. It is just the kind of thinking, moreover, that fuels marginally beneficial treatments (which of course sometimes work, thus encouraging even more of them).

The development in the 1990s, which I think of as the third important change, was the emergence of a small but still growing minority of scientists and others who believe that aging and death can someday be overcome, that they can be treated as diseases like most other medical pathologies. This change is most pronounced in those who believe the average life span can be radically extended and that it would be wrong not to aim for such a goal.[8] Some carry the idea a final step further. The prominent biotechnologist, William Haseltine, CEO of Human Genome Sciences, has declared that "death is nothing but a series of preventable diseases," to be picked off one by one.[9] Although this is a small, but hardy, group of enthusiastic utopians, their influence together with the constant media reporting of important medical breakthroughs, ever hopeful, may be what is strengthening a popular belief among many that medicine can already work miracles, reported increasingly to me anecdotally by many physician colleagues, much to their distress.

I consider this combination of developments over the past 40 years or so a major obstacle to the control of technology (along with an already long list). The first two represent inadvertent, troublesome offshoots of technological progress, neither of which tells against the technology as such, but both of which show how constant innovation has the capacity to muddle our view of death. In neither case was there a belief that, although it can be forestalled, death can be overcome (nor aging either). The third development, part of the movement called "transhumanism," passes beyond muddle into medical utopianism and an accompanying evangelism—the belief that aging and death can be overcome.[10] I consider that movement a social hazard, not only for stimulating what I believe are damaging false hopes by encouraging possibilities that will not be realized in the lifetime of those now in adulthood, if ever. It is no less a social hazard for fueling the engine of technological innovation, elevating its status to a great liberation movement, saving us from our own finite bodies.

Death and the "Full Life"

Death ends our life, but if we have lived a full life, it is hard to know just what of consequence we have been deprived of, or what our fellow citizens have been deprived of by our death. The fact that it would be a delight to add to my long life a visit to Nepal, to learn French, or to go the wedding of my granddaughter, does not mean that, if I cannot work them into the years I have left, I will not have lived a rich and full life even if, at 79, I die tomorrow. George Washington's death after a full life did not deprive our nation of an irreplaceable leader. Others came along to take his place, and it would seem strange to mourn his death now, over 200 years later.

To say this is not to deny that death can be sad and wrenching, an end to our relationship with others, and sometimes with thwarted dreams left over. But that does not prove to me that death is an inherent evil from a long-term perspective. It is just something that goes with the territory of life, a stark territory at times to be sure but one that we can make our way through as earlier generations did. Human life goes on, and the human species has managed to do well enough with the death of individuals, the necessary price of movement and continuing vitality.[11]

Death itself, part of our biological nature, ought not to be seen as the primary target for health care, and particularly when most of us now have the chance to live a full life. The fact that most Americans, some 80% now, will live to old age does not entail, as some seem to think, that we both can and must keep advancing the human life span. Not at all. Compared with all the other evils in the world, the fact that people die in old age should rank near the bottom; and more forestalling of death beyond the present average will add little to our individual or collective lives. The British sociologist John A. Vincent has made a persuasive case that the antiaging movement, especially in its ambition to radically extend life expectancy and to transform the process of aging, actually "devalues old age and older people."[12] The Roman philosopher Seneca wrote that "it is not that we have a short time to live, but that we waste a lot of it. Life is long enough, and a sufficiently generous amount has been given for the highest achievements if it were well-invested. . . . life is long if you know how to use it."[13] He wrote that at a time when average life expectancy was 30 years or so, and old age was taken to arrive at 40.

It is possible to live an adequate and full life in a lesser state of health, particularly if good medical and rehabilitative care can help one adapt to chronic illness and disability. A wonderful feature of human adaptability is the fact that, or so I have observed, the state of a person's health is not a good predictor of a sense of well-being, happiness, or satisfaction with life. We can put up with many ailments well enough. This is of course not true at the outer, nasty edges of illness or disability, which can effectively destroy functional capacity and for which medical care is most needed. But many medical conditions can be tolerated, perhaps lowering the quality of our lives, but by no means destroying it.

THE AMERICAN HEALTH OBSESSION

A peculiarity of the present American health scene is, to over-generalize, that there is an affluent class obsessed with the pursuit of health and many others, usually poorer, who seem indifferent to it or who are unable to pursue it with a similar intensity of the affluent. Fitness clubs, spas, and personal trainers are beyond the reach of most people. The extraordinary interest the media shows in health with every possible danger reported, every possible medical breakthrough cited, and every possible way of reducing health risk detailed plays to the affluent and the educated. They gobble it up. The pursuit of health has, for many, become an obsession and, for even more, an ongoing source of low-level, free-floating anxiety haunted by all those undiagnosed diseases lurking behind our healthy facades. If shopping is a well known therapy for the bored, technological screening has become the best therapy for the worried well: something is out there, or inside of us, waiting to get us; we must catch it early. That pursuit has also had that odd paradoxical feature noted earlier, that the healthier we get, the more worried we get and the more we spend on health. Health care spending in the United States today follows income and affluence, not actual health outcomes.

As Judith Feder and Donald W. Moran have observed, "To be serious about cost containment, it will be necessary to admit that containing costs will require affecting the decisions that individual Americans make every day in all the settings in which they make them."[14] Whether Americans can be brought to think differently about health, to expect less and to settle for less, and to be willing to forgo some health care they might like, or even need, for the sake of the public good, takes a utopian, or maybe a counter-utopian elixir of hope and imagination. I see no plausible alternative.

As individuals, we are in a position similar to our health care system problem. If we do not learn to rein in our aspirations for perfect health, to live with some of our needs that might otherwise be medically dealt with, to run some risks with our health, to understand that an elevated level of this or that reflects a possibility of harm only, not a death sentence, and to recognize (even if begrudgingly) that a cure of one of our otherwise lethal diseases will not save us from some other one. Cured diseases are always succeeded by a final and fatal disease. If we as individuals do not bring some greater realism to our health, some willingness to put up with our mortality and vulnerability, and the anxiety that goes with its recognition, then there is no hope that costs can be controlled, hardly any technologies that can be limited or denied.

There is, to be sure, an obvious objection to my line of thought here. Even if, as individuals, we limit our medical appetite, there is no guarantee that any money saved by our altruism will go to other more serious social or health needs. True enough, and that is one of the serious penalties for living in a society without universal health care and the circumscribed budget that should go with it. But it is also true, as we can see with voting, that it is a bad mistake to think that, with a large electorate, our individual votes are irrelevant. The danger is not that one vote will harm the election process. It is that, if everyone thinks that way, then the process will indeed be harmed. So, if only a few of us begin to change our views of health care, and then a few more, that might indeed make a difference.

My scenario may be fanciful, but the point of this section has been that, as individuals we need an open discussion on what counts as good or bad choices, wise or imprudent ones, and our social obligations to our community as we make them. Such a discussion need not be, and ought not be, coercive. It might, however, help shape some rough consensus, moving us at least in the right direction. There is an obvious truism, usually ignored in health care, that the collective, aggregate impact of our private choices can affect the public good. Hence, it is worth the effort to see if those private choices can be nudged in a helpful direction. That direction would be, following my finite model of health care, toward less, not more, and even much less.

SHAPING A CONSENSUS ON PERSONAL VALUES

A health policy based on a finite set of medical and health policy values and aspirations will look different from the one we now have. It need not be based on the kind of finite model I have offered (other forms are imaginable). But it will have to be built on an understanding that the *ancien régime* of unlimited technological innovation indifferent to costs is over, never to return. It was a regime where health spending was a direct function of national affluence, where health had become a passion for many, where medical research budgets constantly increased, where the media breathlessly proclaimed every new medical advance, where every potential to harm was magnified, where to even question the idea of medical progress was taken as de facto evidence of ludditism and indifference to human suffering, where the best medical care was assumed to be technological care, and where in some quarters the purchase of health care was put in the same category as the purchase of hamburgers, ipods, and plasma TV screens.

It is hard to imagine a cultural setting less congenial to the control of costs or a serious questioning of technology. Infinite aspirations, commercially fed and stimulated, and superintended by the elevation of consumer choice to the highest level, are not a formula for prudent spending or sensible thinking about health needs. If to all of that is harnessed the idea that how we live and how we die, and what we should want in the name of health are, ultimately, personal and self-centered, subject to no restraining ethical or social consensus, no mutual responsibilities, then we are in an exceedingly weak position to formulate meaningful policy.

If we tacitly agree that no one need agree with his fellow citizens on such intimate matters as how much and what kind of health to seek, then we will be left with two harsh alternatives. One of them will be imposed rationing, overriding what we may want—which we have been tutored to believe is no one's business but our own—and that will seem arbitrary and authoritarian. The other will be a triumph of the kind of consumer-directed health care meant to force us to think how much we are willing to spend, both giving us choice and forcing us to use it, and will leave us by the wayside if we are unwilling or unable to bankrupt ourselves or our families to buy it. The only way to avoid such harsh outcomes in a financially stressed health care system is to see if a consensus, even if a rough one, can be achieved, one that simultaneously provides reasonably good health care but also imposes acceptable limits on what we ought to want.

If there is plenty of money to go around, it may not matter much whether we have a consensus or not because all tastes, desires, and inclinations can be satisfied; and that is what most Americans have had until recently. But if budgets become tight, then some agreement is necessary. The increase in chronic and degenerative disease adds a growing impetus. They are changing health care needs and demands while at the same time generating a whole new and difficult range of medical choices. In essence, they manifest a decline in acute illnesses, putting in their place a slow decline that can require expensive technologies over a long time to preserve life, often with only marginal benefits. The patients cannot be cured, but they can be treated, their diseases managed until they die.

Death is the final outcome, but it now arrives at a slow and leisurely pace. If the extended life is often seen as a benefit, the extended pressure on physicians and family caretakers is not. A sudden heart attack was a shock to families, but death was over and done with in a hurry. Congestive heart failure, slowly going downhill but fluctuating from day to day, and with considerable and erratic patient pain and discomfort and protracted family anxiety, is a far more subtle problem to deal with.[15]

A variety of concepts, influential and widely used in patient care and policy decisions, and in the criteria for insurance benefits need a new focus, one that works to achieve a usable consensus for treating individuals in the face of the new medical situation. They are "medical necessity," "reasonable and necessary," and "cost effectiveness," which I approach in this chapter from the perspective of individuals. In the next chapter I discuss what constitutes a reasonable "basic package" or "decent minimum" of care and return to "cost effectiveness," but from a population perspective.

MEDICAL NECESSITY, REASONABLE AND NECESSARY

Insurers, government agencies, and physicians must determine what constitutes acceptable medical diagnosis and treatment. The terms "medical necessity" and "reasonable and necessary" (used more or less interchangeably) have historically played a central role in such determinations. In earlier decades there was no such language. Physicians were free to treat patients as they saw fit as long as their practices were "appropriate" and met a "community standard." Those latter standards were vague, and not by accident. Their aim was not to impose rules or standards with any serious bite on the doctor–patient relationship. That relationship was a not a two-way street, with doctors and patients negotiating a treatment plan. Physicians decided, and patients were expected to follow the "doctors orders" (a phrase that still had currency into the 1960s).

Much has changed in recent years, driven in great part by both cost and quality considerations as well as improved administrative rationality and consistency. Although they are often hard to distinguish in practice, there is a difference between making a solely patient-oriented treatment decision, the classical individual patient welfare standard, and a policy decision focused on population benefits, which may override individual patient welfare. My discussion in this chapter focuses on patient-oriented decisions.

The Social Security Act says that Medicare will not cover services that are "not reasonable and necessary for the diagnosis or treatment of illness or injury or to improve the functioning of a mal-formed body member."[16] Although this standard is widely used and is workable with many common medical situations, it has proved to be too vague to deal with the complexities of technological developments, on one hand, and changing social and cultural standards, on the other. "Insurers," one useful study concluded (and consistent with others) "have largely abandoned their direct attempts to limit the utilization rate for most medical procedures."[17] Again and again the insurers have lost in courts when claims against them for treatment denials in the name of medical necessity were granted as if judges have simply capitulated to doctor–patient decisions. There are many reasons why those efforts failed, but Mark Hall's judgment that "it reflects broader social and professional antipathy to medical decisions being made by anyone other than the affected patient and treating decisions," seems just right.[18]

Yet that de facto return to the older standard almost surely reflects the permissive, physician-dominated medically relativistic culture I described above. A long-standing goal in the use of medical necessity as a standard has been to pursue both quality and cost control together, as if those are compatible ends. That seems to me plausible only if one limits the scope of "quality" to essentially technical considerations, that of the medical benefits of the treatment outcomes. Does a treatment do what it is intended to do—save life, restore physical or mental functioning, relieve pain, and so on?

But "quality" in an affluent society covers many connotations not well caught by narrow technical standards. The combination of an inflated notion of patient self-definition and the infinity model of technological innovation guarantees the failure of "medical necessity" to be of much use. If to that combination is added a resistance to taking cost into account as an acceptable basis for decisions, then the door is left wide open for cost escalation.

PATIENT SELF-DEFINITION

I use the phrase "patient self-definition" to capture an idea that is not quite identical with "patient self-determination." It is widely agreed that, as in end-of-life care, patient self-determination is a moral right, generally interpreted to mean a right to say no to treatment or to terminate it once started. A more complicated, and increasingly common, situation arises when a patient wants some treatment that, in the eyes of her physician, is useless, potentially harmful, or outside the scope of standard medical practice. Patients frequently win those struggles, in great part because of a deference to patient self-definition, that is, the presumption that, however strange it may seem to others, patients have a positive right to direct their own lives and set their own medical goals, not simply the right to say no to unwanted treatments.

There are at least two major instances where the right of self-definition has a clinical impact. First, the notion of "quality" increasingly goes well beyond technical considerations. Affluent societies raise the level and scope of an acceptable quality for just about anything and every thing to an ever higher level. What we now count as a decent quality automobile, as with medical care, encompasses a steadily growing list of amenity features: better radios and GPR devices, quieter, improved safety features, and higher horsepower. Where once most of those features were optional, they are now standard (with a corresponding increase in cost); and the innovation with them continues apace.

For Americans, good quality health care encompasses improved amenities (single-bed hospital rooms, up-to-date TV sets and telephones, and good food), improved services (no waiting time), and the latest and best technology. Most of those items do not affect health outcomes in any significant way, any more than better auto audio systems or higher horsepower is likely to get us from point A to B any better than in the past, but they do guarantee an increase in cost.

The second notion of "quality" I define as "marginal benefit." This concept has many dimensions. This year's new model auto is much the same as last year's, but the advertisements will let us know that many small improvements have been made and new features added. An analogous move is visible in the response of the pharmaceutical industry to charges that many so-called new drugs are little more than me-too drugs. Their response is that, although there may be only a little chemical difference between new drug X and old drug Y, it is just that difference that may allow a physician to find a drug that is not merely "good enough" for a patient but exactly "the right" drug. The patient gain will likely be marginal, but the cost difference significant. Marginal benefit also has a role in difficult medical decisions, for instance, that of a low probability (but much desired) outcome at a high cost (e.g., beneficial for only 5% of patients). If patient self-definition is allowed to rule, then the notion of "benefit" is strictly for the patient to determine and will be helped along by a physician who believes that individual patient benefit and physician judgment trump all other values.

One of the most striking efforts to give some binding substance to the concept of "medical necessity" was published in 1996, the outcome of a workshop sponsored by the National Institute for Health Care Management, and led by the economist-physician David M. Eddy.[19] The aim was to develop "coverage criteria" for insurers and for designing benefit language. It was acknowledged that no criteria could be perfect, could deal with all ambiguities, and could "prevent patients, providers or plans from subverting the criteria's objectives." But the criteria Eddy and his colleagues developed are as important now as they were over a decade ago—but also as neglected:

- The intervention is used for a medical condition.
- There is sufficient evidence to draw conclusions about the intervention's effects on health outcomes.
- The evidence demonstrates that the intervention can be expected to produce its intended effects on health outcomes.
- The intervention's expected beneficial effects on health outcomes outweigh its expected harmful effects.
- The intervention is the most cost-effective method available to address the medical conditions.

Each of the criteria was accompanied by definitions, only two of which I cite here. "Medical condition: a medical condition is a disease, or illness, or an injury. A biological or psychological condition that lies within the range of normal human variation is not considered a disease, illness, or injury."[20] "Health outcomes: health outcomes are outcomes of medical conditions that directly affect the length or quality of a person's life."

Those criteria, as I am sure Eddy and his colleagues would agree, can be interpreted in an infinite or finite direction (to use my earlier categories). A finite direction would (in my view), for instance, eliminate coverage for contraceptives, male or female (because a risk of pregnancy from intercourse is not a disease, illness, or injury); for assisted reproduction for women over the age of 35 (because a decline in fertility beyond that age is not a disease or illness either); for erectile dysfunction for men over the age of 65 (a normal pattern, not a disease); repeat joint or other surgery for men and women who, after the age of 65, want to continue an athletic recreational life (joint problems increase with age and are not necessarily a disease); a denial of screening of people for low probability diseases unless there is a clear family history of risk; denial of mental health coverage for all but the most severe cases, not as a response to an unhappy life, a troubled romance, or difficulties raising one's children.

That list could be continued at much greater length, but my rule for a finite health care would be to place a heavy burden on patients and their physicians to justify medical care. I should ask myself: am I really sick, or really threatened, with a preventable illness? Can I tolerate some minor pain and inconvenience? My physician should be asking comparable questions when I present myself. The standard for answering such questions should be narrowly medical and the required outcome one that "directly in some substantial way affects the length or quality of a person's life." A relief of anxiety that one might be sick, or might be at risk, should invoke the burden-of-proof principle: no screening or treatment without established symptoms or long-term, verifiable threats; health anxieties, unless clinically extreme and strongly plausible, should not count.

As for treatment, patients should not be given any that do not meet the "sufficient evidence" standard, based on well-controlled clinical trials, or, if nonetheless prescribed, patients should be fully informed about the absence of such trials and the alternative method of evaluation being used by their physicians. "How do you know your proposed treatment will do me any good?" Patient education programs to know how to ask such questions and evaluate the answers would be appropriate. In general, the rule for patients should be: do not go to your doctor in the absence of symptoms (save for those conditions directly reflecting the pathologies of aging or family histories of particular diseases), do not be screened for any but likely pathologies, and serious ones at that, and do not accept treatment without the likelihood of a good outcome (a standard of "it might help" or "it would not hurt to try" would not be good enough). One obvious complication, of course, is that even if a treatment has passed the test of solid clinical research, there is no guarantee if will work equally well with all patients. Uncertainty is always a part of treatment decisions.

Medical necessity, however, has always connoted black-and-white choices: a treatment is either necessary or it is not. But the terms "necessary" and "necessity" could well be broken down into more nuanced gradations. The present standard, in effect, opens the way for a wide range of procedures and treatments that can usefully be distinguished, and for which different working norms can be devised. It would be useful, in short, to return to an effort too quickly abandoned, that of establishing a hierarchical range of procedures and treatments, which could be used administratively to set fiscal priorities and clinically to establish relative urgency, thus making room for increased or reduced co-payments and policy decisions. Here is a possible system, adapted from a variety of U.S. and foreign efforts in the late 1980s and 1990s. I list them in a rough order of priority and have in mind only the making of individual clinical conditions:

- Acute, life-threatening illnesses (heart attacks, stroke, appendicitis)
- Long-term lethal chronic and degenerative diseases (cancer, diabetes, heart and kidney failure, Alzheimer disease)
- Long-term nonlethal but life-shortening, disease (severe mental illness, Parkinson's disease, COPD)
- Less severe long-term, controllable nonlethal conditions (milder mental illness, frailty)
- Conditions amenable to rehabilitation (injuries from accidents, stroke)
- Borderline cases: medical care for reasons other than disease and injury (athletic impairments, infertility treatment for young adults)

MEDICAL NECESSITY: A CLINICAL PERSPECTIVE

In sum, and in keeping with the finite model I developed above, medical necessity from a clinical perspective would be to provide a level of care for individuals that enabled them to go from being a young person to being an old person, and to do so with a quality of life necessary for them to pursue personal, family, and work roles. But there would be no expectation of perfection, and indeed, an expectation that some degree of pain and anxiety would have to be endured.

A finite model of health care requires a finite, closed-end budget to make any policy sense. Of course in a health-obsessed society, the budget could be set at a very high level, but to do so would threaten other important social goods. A health budget in such a society would have to be set in a way that it would not trump most other social spending, which it now does in our society. One point is evident from the outset: with little dissent, a wide range of analysts and commentators have said in recent years that "medically reasonable and necessary" as a treatment standard is much too vague to have any serious impact on costs. Such a definition can work reasonably well with solidly established therapies to treat well-established medical conditions based on well-grounded evidence. Where it does not work is for new therapies with marginal benefits or in the use of older therapies with a low probability of success. And it will be useful only if to "medical necessity" or "reasonable and necessary" is added "cost effective."

That additional condition has been and will doubtless remain an uphill struggle. An important reason why managed care stopped cost escalation for a time in the mid-1990s was that it made some use of EBM, cost-effectiveness analysis, required the use of primary care physicians as gatekeepers for access to specialists, and required physicians to gain approval for the use of expensive technologies or those of uncertain medical value. That was just the right combination to control costs effectively, and it worked remarkably well for a time (although helped by insurers artificially holding premiums down for a short-term competitive advantage). That was just the wrong combination politically. Patients and physicians revolted at their restrictions, and legislatures had no hesitation to mandate treatments that ignored evidence against them, caving in to public or interest group pressure.[21] That history, together with the story of the demise of the 1979–1981 National Center for Health Care Technology Assessment (chapter 5), the OTA, and the neutering of the HCPR stand out in my mind as three depressing stories about efforts to assess technology and take cost control seriously. They were good ideas, and still are, and require another try.

The HMO failure in the mid-1990s indicates the profound resistance of patients and doctors to interference with autonomy, even when it is a strong, collective benefit to the healthcare system. Physician and industry resistance to technology assessment reflects a long tradition of physician hostility to outside interference as does market-driven resistance to government control. One could hardly find better examples of the power of culture, different cultures in each case, but all of them well-entrenched in our national health care psyche.

Sean Tunis, a former high level official with the CMS and an astute technology analyst, has noted three obstacles to change in the resistance to technology assessment: a lack of stakeholder confidence in just about any decision-making process, undercutting the acceptance of any possible consensus; resistance to any entity other than physicians and patients making clinical decisions; and worries that any serious cost criteria for Medicare decisions will have a negative impact on innovation.[22] To this intimidating list may be added industry resistance and the widely held belief that it is simply immoral to put a price on human life. Nonetheless, although well aware of the myriad sources of resistance, Peter Neumann and other distinguished analysts have said that "Medicare's policy of paying for any medical advance that has positive benefits, regardless of its costs, is unsustainable."[23] Jacqueline Fox, a legal scholar who has written a masterful study of the Congressional resistance to cost considerations, has underlined the deepest problem, a total unwillingness to take on "extremely expensive, medically effective technology."[24]

The Harvard geriatrician Muriel Gillick analyzed three Medicare decisions to provide coverage for expensive technologies: lung-volume reduction surgery, implantable cardioverter-defibrillators, and left ventricular assist devices. Their aggregate costs can add between $1 billion and $7 billion to the annual Medicare budget. Yet only one of them scores well in the ratio of costs to quality-adjusted life years, that of the defibrillator, a standard that, in any case, was not actually used to assess the three new technologies.[25] Moreover, most of the benefits of the three technologies, even when successful, can be judged marginal in their benefits. Clinical trials on lung-reduction surgery brought a 16% improvement in exercise capacity, compared with 3% for those treated medically. The cardioverter–defibrillators allowed a 6% decrease in risk of death, but had a higher risk of hospitalization for heart failure than those treated medically. For the left ventricular assist devices, the survival rate was only 52% at 1 year and 23% at 2 years.

The Medicare Coverage Advisory Committee voted to support all three technologies, saying of one of them that it offered "substantial benefit to patients with severe congestive heart failure."[26] Substantial? Those figures indicate a soft notion of "substantial," but one compatible with a self-definition of substantial, one in which relatively poor results are legitimized. Peter J. Neumann and his colleagues examined Medicare coverage decisions from 1999 to 2007 and concluded that about 60% of its favorable decisions were based on evidence "no better than fair," though often with conditions placed on coverage.[27]

A "NEGATIVE IMPACT ON INNOVATION"?

As I have noted earlier in this book, a fear that controls on technological innovation would dampen innovation turns out to be a crucial variable, itself dampening efforts to control its costs. "There is," Sean Tunis has written, "a justifiable concern that the [CMS] decision-making process may have a considerable effect on the overall economic vitality of the pharmaceutical, biotechnology, and medical device industries. . . . the availability of investment capital for medical technology might be affected, perhaps resulting in fewer forms of technology, losses in employment, and reduced exports."[28]

Perhaps those dire prospects would turn out to be true. But if most if not all efforts to seriously control technology cost are failing, and likely at the present pace of reform to continue failing, then it would seem utterly naïve, if not foolish, to worry about reduced innovation and industry losses. That is precisely what we should hope for. We cannot both hope to better manage technology costs and yet, at the same time, bemoan the possibility that it might work. It is as if we told an alcoholic that he should stop drinking, but that it would be wrong not to set before him all the interesting new drinks being developed, some of which his alcoholism might tolerate. Cost reduction will require fewer new technologies, especially those with marginal benefits, slower diffusion of expensive ones, a reduced dependence upon technology by physicians, and a willingness of patients to change their expectations and lower their demands.

"Policymaking," Tunis continues, "should focus on getting good value from health care spending. At a minimum, there should be public dialogue about how to ensure a high quality and safe health care that gives patients freedom of choice in making health care decisions, expands access to care, encourages innovation, and is affordable."[29] But do the figures on the three technologies cited by Gillick represent a "good value," the kind of innovation that should be encouraged, and are they affordable? I would say they have none of those features. As a symbol of the technological problem with the kind of chronic conditions they are meant to treat, arresting a lethal downward decline for a relatively short time at a high cost, they hardly represent "substantial benefit." But it is currently irrelevant what I, or anyone other than doctor and patient, take to be a benefit—if we want it, we can usually have it. That is what freedom of choice means.

Even so, should not doctors and their patients have the freedom to choose the latest technological procedures even if their benefits are marginal? There will surely be many patients who will choose them, and many physicians who will recommend them to desperate patients. Who are we, the well, to say that such a choice is wrong or to decide for others what is a good and bad reason for making a life-saving choice? A 23% 2-year survival rate for cardioverter-defibrillators is, many would say, better than a 0% rate. I do not commend the situation I have just described, but I think the description is accurate.

There is no consensus about such choices at the individual patient level nor are there any efforts even to have a "public dialogue" about them; and many would probably find such a dialogue morally offensive as, after all, no price tag, it is said, can be put on the value of a human life. Nonetheless, how we *ought* to make our personal choices needs to be pushed into a public dialogue, however awkward and stressful that dialogue might be at times. No one would object to dialogue on the topics as defined by Tunis, all of which are triumphs of positive thinking: the discussion would just not be enough or sufficiently probing—something I am sorry to say because Sean Tunis has done wonderful work in opening up the cost-effectiveness debate.

Although I hope people will increasingly not choose to be treated with expensive technologies that have a marginal benefit only (as I think the case with Gillick's three technologies), it would be a mistake to assume such a development or to base policy on it. Instead, the dialogue should be twofold: whether and to what extent and at what costs we as individuals should want technological medicine if available to us, and what technologies should be available for such choices. The former will be a personal decision, the latter a social decision. If a treatment is available as a standard part of Medicare coverage, patients cannot be denied what will be an established benefit entitlement. That door will have to remain open, but the standards for entitlement can be raised, closing the door bit by bit.

Alternatively, because of their cost, a very high co-payment could be required, at a level to make even the desperate think twice (e.g., 50% of the costs). But that requirement would be a cruel form of consumer-directed health care, the kind designed to give people choices but also to make them think seriously, and even desperately, about making them, and all the more so if the choice is life or death or sustained misery. The only feasible alternative left is simply not to make the technology available or, if it is already available, not to allow it to be chosen unless the particular case passes the "sufficient evidence" test proposed by Dr. Eddy and his colleagues.

Even then, David Eddy's standards leave us with a problem. Let us imagine that, for a particular treatment, all of his standards but one have been met. His last standard is where the rub comes: "the intervention is the most cost-effective method available to address the medical conditions." But that method could be outrageously expensive, the provision of which would seem to be, and would be, unfair to the less expensive, equally beneficial needs of others. In short, there may well be situations, particularly as expensive technologies are improved to meet the other standards, where money will painfully poke us in our financial eye. The greatest problem in the long run will be with our technological successes, not our failures, wonderfully effective, yet horribly costly.

The debate on the use of cost effectiveness criteria has arisen precisely to deal with the problem of the availability of technologies; and thus indirectly, whether patients should be able to choose them at public expense. Congress has refused to allow cost to be considered in Medicare coverage decisions, and with the exception of specific exclusions in health insurance contracts, the private sector will follow this lead. But let us assume that Congress might someday, shortly one hopes, allow cost as a consideration. How valuable and robust are the available tools for doing so? They come down to three possibilities: the use of cost effectiveness and cost–benefit criteria, value-for-money standards, and the use of democratically organized committees and group mechanisms to make decisions.

HOW EFFECTIVE IS A
COST-EFFECTIVENESS STANDARD?

When Congress has been urged, unsuccessfully, to allow cost as a consideration in Medicare decisions, the method usually invoked to do so is "cost effectiveness." A full standard of judgment for a new therapy, treatment, or device would then be "reasonable, necessary, and cost effective." But would "cost effectiveness" make any real difference? There is reason to have some doubts about that, in part because of some ambiguity in the meaning of the term.

There are two meanings in use. One of them is that a treatment "is as effective as an alternative but less expensive,"[30] or, as David Eddy put it "an intervention is considered cost effective if there is no other available intervention that offers a clinically appropriate benefit at a lower cost."[31] Muriel Gillick has a different definition: "cost effectiveness analysis considers the marginal cost of a new procedure for each quality-adjusted year of life that a patient gains."[32] The phrase "value for money" or something similar often appears in the cost-effectiveness literature as well.

Jacqueline Fox, although citing a conventional definition, goes on immediately to note that "if no alternative technology exists, any effectiveness is cost-effective."[33] That shrewd observation (self-evident but rarely mentioned) means, in effect, that cost effectiveness can be meaningfully used only when the "new treatment" can be compared with an older treatment for the same condition; otherwise it is useless. Nonetheless, a new technology that offers any benefit may well be adopted because it offers some hope in the absence of an alternative.

She also notes, however, that in 1989 CMS proposed criteria for coverage decisions that went well beyond "effectiveness," including "indirect costs such as increased productivity of the disabled and various transportation costs. These would be given a monetary value for purposes of the coverage decision evaluation."[34] That proposal got nowhere but was in effect a cost–benefit proposal, one seeking "to determine if the cost of paying for something is worth the benefit to society based on the society's valuation of both the benefit and the cost."[35] On that point (what QALYs are meant to do) she goes on to observe that, in moving away from a softer cost-effectiveness standard and toward cost–benefit calculations, "the more it seeks to have cost-effectiveness accomplish, the more they risk confrontation over their decisions."[36]

Peter Neumann and his colleagues add a further twist. "Cost-effective analysis is not a cost-containment tool but, rather, a technique to improve value."[37] At the same time they say that cost-effectiveness analysis "could save money," but such saving would depend on the thresholds and aggressiveness that policy-makers apply. They then go on, much to my surprise, to present a QALYs table showing the "cost-effectiveness" of various medical interventions (cost/QALY); that is, they end up using a cost–benefit standard that they have labeled cost effectiveness.[38] The net result is a threefold confusing mixture, stirred into the same pot: cost effectiveness, cost–benefit, and improvement of value.

I have tried to look carefully at the various terms used to provide tools for controlling costs and, in particular, the cost of old and new technologies. The variant definitions and usages—themselves failing to provide a consensus even among the experts, all of whom are grappling with the cost problem—do not provide an encouraging prospect. If this problem poses dilemmas in the fashioning of generalized policy, where the common good must be pursued, it becomes all the more acute at the doctor–patient level, when there is (at present) only the individual patient good to be considered. Cost-effectiveness analysis will be of no use with an entirely new technology, with nothing available for comparison. Value for money as a criterion seems hardly more useful. If patient self-definition is the de facto rule-of-thumb, only the patient can decide what counts as a value, and for some patients a 100 to 1 chance of a good outcome at a high cost is better than the "zero value" of being dead. As long as some expensive treatments are available, even with low probability outcomes, some patients, even many, are likely to want them; and doctors have no principled way of saying no.

Despite all of these technical and political difficulties, cost–benefit analysis making use of QALYs seems to me the most plausible technical solution to the individual treatment problem, certainly the best among a weak lot. But my analysis in general leads me to think that, in our self-definition culture, there is not now and will never be a satisfactory technical solution, much less one that will pass political muster. There is no way to look at a cost number by itself, however large, and to say it is "too much." "Compared with what, and under what circumstances?" would be the appropriate rejoinder to an objection. If we can afford to pay star athletes multimillion dollar salaries, and fund a multibillion dollar war in Iraq, surely we can spend that kind of money to save lives. Right?

Everything will depend on context, and in our open-ended health care system, one with no budget limits, one that conflates technological aggressiveness and the sanctity of life and allows each of us to make our own decision about value, there is no meaningful context to do that. No legislator is likely to support openly a treatment standard that will ration care to particular, identifiable patients, or one where high cost alone is the decisive test, or one that excessively depends on an impersonal economic calculation.

I have painted myself into a corner, rejecting or belittling one possible approach after another in making technological decisions for individual care. But because one of the aims of this book is to cut through outright denial of the technology cost problem (the path taken by Congress and Medicare) and to examine assorted tactical approaches, inspired by hope and desperation, to see if they might actually work in some decisive way, I cannot feel too guilty. It is hard to fine good technical and political solutions for problems deeply rooted in our culture and politics.

How do we get an affluent, individualistic culture, one economically profligate in so many ways, yet incredibly tight-fisted in others (e.g., taxes), and in love with technology of all kinds, to change its ways? A finite model of health care will require a change of personal values, but that is unlikely to happen without a finite health care system based on a different set of values, themselves finite in their thrust. If, as I have argued, we will not find good formulas in our culture, economically or politically, to deal with individual cases, is there a policy approach that might work? Other than screaming warnings at ourselves, is there some way of organizing our house to overcome the demonstrated fact that our beloved pet is out of control, resistant to the best of trainers? That question is the topic of the next chapter.

CHAPTER 7

⊗

REDEFINING "MEDICAL NECESSITY"

FROM INDIVIDUAL GOOD TO SOCIAL GOOD

"Medical necessity" has not worked well in practice as a standard of care for individuals and is all but useless in dealing with costly technologies. The concept runs up against three confounding elements. One of these is the force of medicalization, which over time turns many desires into felt needs, particularly as medical progress finds ways to treat undesirable pathological conditions that were earlier simply taken to be an unavoidable part of life. Another is that of using medical means to deal with problems that are not inherently medical at all but are amenable to medical solutions (the contraceptive pill to avoid pregnancy; cosmetic surgery to improve appearance). Still another is the wide, intractable range of opinion and belief about acceptable qualities of life and individual functioning, a range bolstered by a deep-seated belief in the right of self-definition and physician judgment. The result of these three elements working together is that "medical necessity" cannot be given a standardized, acceptable meaning, one generally viable either for treatment decisions or technology coverage.

If the notion of medical necessity for individuals cannot work, but some useful concept is needed, is there an alternative? A concept of necessity that blends individual and population benefit may do so. What fails as a useful standard for individuals can work much better in evaluating the health of populations. What is medically necessary for the health of a society is not the same as for the health of individuals. There are many things I would define as a necessity for my life, but a failure to provide them, although it might hurt or diminish me personally, might not negatively affect my society. If we think that the only standard of importance in a health care system is the good of individuals, and that good is solely between them and their physicians to decide (the irreducible ethical core of traditional medicine), then the notion of a societal good is ruled out from the start, and with it the possibility of controlling costs.

We have, however, customarily made an exception for matters labeled "public health," which focuses on population health (control of contagious disease, sanitation and good water, disease prevention, immunization, health surveillance) and can in its name restrict individual liberties. We can adapt that model, I contend, with some pertinent alterations, to the provision of health care and the assessment of technology. Instead of thinking about medical care in terms of individual benefits, why not adapt public health modes of thinking to individual patient care?

I would put the question I want to pursue this way: which policies for the provision of treatment and the use of technology will do the most good from a population, not individual perspective? If agreement can be reached on that point, then the foundation will have been laid for a health care system that can much better control costs. To pursue that question I make use of a number of ingredients.

First, I argue that, as a general proposition, the United States, along with most other developed countries, already has sufficient good health to function well economically and socially. It need not indefinitely improve average life expectancy, already adequate, but there is considerable room for an improvement in the quality of life, in removing gross inequities affecting various subgroups, and in dealing with some new problems of childhood health (e.g., obesity). Second, I propose that health care ought not be approached solely in terms of the needs and treatment of individuals, but primarily, even if not exclusively, from a population, common good, perspective. Third, I lay out a number of premises of a strategy for cost control, each meant to embody a population-based strategy. Fourth, I propose a set of levels of health care that statistically move from the most common medical needs to the less common, and offer that statistical strategy as a tool for policymaking. Fifth, I sketch a way of developing an affordable, sustainable basic package of health care for each age group.

Do we really have any choice about going in the direction of population-based care? We are trapped. If no successful individual standard of medical necessity can be devised, then we must look elsewhere, toward a population health standard. Readers with a philosophical bent will immediately sniff out a "common good" principle, and they will be correct. Used with care, and blended with sensitivity to individual needs, it is the best available principle for making policy decisions, although it is one which may often, in the name of fiscal responsibility and sustainability, require putting individual interests in a secondary position.

PREMISES OF A POPULATION-BASED HEALTH POLICY

Here is a question rarely asked: just how healthy must a population be in order to have a well-functioning, reasonably happy, economically viable, and just society? We know from the experience of sub-Saharan countries how deadly is HIV disease, not simply because it kills many but because it kills those younger people who are responsible for raising families and maintaining the infrastructure of society; and it leaves millions of children orphans. We know also, at the other end of the spectrum, that developed countries can thrive despite high death rates, now mainly in old age, and with a fair amount of illness and disability in its younger population. At the same time, in otherwise healthy countries, various minorities and subgroups can have death rates and health status well below the average (as with black males), and that is unacceptable.

Is a society such as ours, in which the majority of us die in old age (some 80% after the age of 65 in the United States), to be accounted an unhealthy *society*? I think not, if mortality rates alone are to be the test. By that standard we are the healthiest people with the greatest life expectancy in American history. But what about all the other injuries and diseases that afflict all age groups as well as all the elderly people who are suffering from chronic and degenerative diseases and going slowly and painfully downhill to their deaths? They can quite fairly be said to be unhealthy and limited in their capacity to direct their own lives as they might wish.

But the existence of these groups, to which we will all belong at one point or another in our lives, does not show that, generally speaking, we can characterize our society as unhealthy. If the existence of aged ill is the test, there never will, or could be, a "healthy" society. Nor can it be said, with the exception of the poor, that bad health as such is a national problem, a major domestic issue doing harm to our economic, educational, and social life. The high cost of caring for the sick is a national problem, but that is because we have chosen, as a society, to provide expensive health care; however, that is an entirely different matter from saying that illness and death per se are a serious problem at the present level of American health. There is no moral obligation or imperative to continually improve the general health of populations already at historic high levels. But we can, and should, work to improve the health of those who are at much lower levels, bringing them up to the levels of those with a long life expectancy and a decent quality of health.

Two economic perspectives bear out that last observation. One of them is, as Thomas E. Getzen has written, "that the amount spent on health care is determined by the amount available to spend rather than the amount of disease is obvious, but has not always been consistently incorporated in discussions of health policy."[1] Getzen answers the question implicit in the title of his article "Health Care as an Individual Necessity or a National Luxury?" by saying it is both. We spend much money on health and on medical technology because it is available to spend, and while we have long complained about high costs and the dangers they pose, that does not much deter us from spending more, all in the name of the expanding circle of need and necessity. Needs (what we as individuals find desirable mentally or physically) are expanded by medicalization and available technology to necessities, but neither shows that, as a country, we really need all we *think* we need or that every need is truly a necessity.

A distinguished Spanish economist Guillem Lopez has argued that "increasing health care expenditures does not in fact have a significant impact on life expectancy or most of the conventional health indicators, other perhaps than those related to quality aspects. . . . given that in most developed countries we observe decreasing marginal benefits from additional expenditures on life and death outputs, [their government] finance seems less justifiable."[2] If then, as discussed in chapter 3, ever more medical technology does not commensurately generate better overall health, nor do higher medical expenditures necessarily improve health to more than a modest degree, there is no good policy reason for tolerating rising costs. And they should not be tolerated merely because they create serious economic problems but also because they are represent a waste or money, are of little use to our health, and indeed, are often harmful to it. The high cost of marginal population health benefits, that gap between what we spend and what we get for our money, makes rising health care costs truly a luxury.

One hundred years ago, before the great improvement in health, one could have made a case that our country was economically harmed by illness and death. The vigorous effort to carry out medical research and improved health care made an enormous difference. But now that we have a high level of health, one sufficient to carry the country along, there is no longer a societal need for indefinite, endless improvement. For the sake of relieving individual suffering, it is a civic good to work for improvement, but it is no longer a civic necessity. The necessity, by contrast, lies in helping everyone to achieve the health status enjoyed by the healthiest, reducing inequities in care, and doing so in an affordable way, which means an end to an obsession with raising everyone's health status regardless of cost or competing national needs. Hardly less important is the need to eliminate the economic anxiety that illness incurs for millions of Americans. It is bad enough to put up with illness physically and psychologically without the added burden of worrying how to pay for treatment.

If we use the unlimited progress and innovation ideal as our model, and apply it to everyone who is sick, then one could say that illness, pain, suffering, and death are widespread and thus ought to be eliminated or their effects ameliorated as far as possible. But that ideal, applied as it commonly is to individuals, does not show that our society—our common life together—is threatened in any basic way. We know that poverty increases the likelihood of illness and disease, but it is the poverty that is the real enemy here and only secondarily the health of the poor. We know also that unemployment is correlated with poor health, but it is the lack of jobs not the health consequences that constitutes the core issue. None of our major domestic or international problems are caused by bad health: global warming, the terrorist threat, crime and domestic violence, the international trade deficit, major income disparities, broken marriages and families, poverty, immigration troubles, and racism.

In many of those cases, it is easy to see a deleterious health impact, but they are a consequence of harmful social conditions, not the cause. To be sure, sick people can reduce a nation's productivity. They may not be able to work or work well below their capacity. Yet I have never heard a plausible argument, much less evidence, that the loss of productivity by the sick is a serious threat to our economy.

As one who has long espoused the European idea of solidarity as a far better moral foundation for the provision of health care than an individualistic appeal to justice or rights, what I am advocating may seem odd and inconsistent. I understand solidarity to be a view of community that takes the provision of health care to rest on mutual empathy in the face of illness and on reciprocal obligations to provide care to each other to reduce our common suffering. But that shared value does not relieve us of the need to determine how far, and in what ways, we should go to provide care and to determine what kind of care is most appropriate. Nor does it entail that any and all human suffering brought on by illness must be relieved to the last jot and title. "Less is more" can apply as well in health care as in many other areas of life.

By emphasizing the societal effect of poor health, not just its individual burdens, I am proposing a different way of looking at health (limiting its value as one human good among many, not trumping others) and thus of health care (from an infinite to a finite model). This view does not negate the solidarity we should feel for our neighbor, but it does push us to ask just what kind of effect our poor health may have on other common civic problems; and that may be less than we think. Such a view may also help us to take a more perceptive look at the excessively high status of health and health care in America. It is easier to find money to deal with the health fallout of poverty (e.g., Medicaid) than to deal with the problem directly.

SOME NECESSARY PREMISES

Based on the finite model of health care presented in the previous chapter, I now suggest some specific premises, or principles, of a finite population-based health policy. From there, I move to the use of age-based categories for the allocation of resources.

"Medical Necessity" as a Social Norm

Here is my formal definition of "medical necessity" as a social and not individual norm. A medical treatment and the use of a technology is medically necessary when its use will have benefits for (1) an entire population, or (2) some significant and identifiable subgroup of the population, and for (3) some individual patients as well. If category 3 cannot show any gain for categories 1 and 2, then it should have a reduced claim to resources. The pertinent categories I now offer in making such assessments will be by age groupings and by proposing some categories for setting health care priorities, but with special provision for minority groups. The use of QALYs will be a principal means of determining benefits but softened by leaving open the way for other considerations, including age.

A population–common good approach takes the good of the community as its highest standard, making room for individual needs but not letting these trump common goods, or only rarely. It does not use disease categories as its starting point but puts them in a secondary position as well. The decisionmaking process for providing treatment would move through three steps. In approving a new device to combat heart disease, for instance, it would be necessary to determine (1) what its value would be for different age groups, (2) what it would cost to provide it to each age group, (3) what would be the health benefits in terms of QALYs for each age group in enhancing the possibility of a full life span. Approval would be granted only if good answers could be given to these questions. What about orphan diseases and treatments for those conditions that affect comparatively few group members? I will return to that crucial difficult question later, after I have developed my population-approach further.

Achieving a Full, Not Endless, Life

The most important aim of a health care system should be to help a person go from being a young person to becoming an old person. However, once a person has achieved that goal, there ought to be a reduced obligation on the part of a health care system to help someone become indefinitely older, much less as old as that person might like. A full life, I believe, can be achieved by most people sometime between the ages of 70 and 80, and the health care system should aim to make the years between birth and that age range its main goal. After age 80, which is the outer (but not inflexible) limit for policy purpose, the priority should shift from the cure of disease and acute care medicine to the provision of good long-term and home care, together with solid rehabilitation and income support. As it presently happens, acute care costs for the elderly decline after age 80, but it is reasonable to expect that these costs will rise with a (likely) more demanding patient baby boom population.

In an earlier book, I spoke of a "natural life span," suggesting the late 70s or early 80s as the time when most people would have achieved such a span.[3] Well, the word "natural" brings out hives in some people, and it was commonly noted that, with increasingly extended life expectancies, there is no biologically fixed length of life and thus no "natural" life span.[4] The notion of a "full life" better captures what I was trying to say. It is a phrase that I have frequently heard used to describe the breadth of experience that an elderly person has had by the end of life. I take it to mean that someone has had the chance to live a life long enough to enjoy most, although not necessarily all, of the pleasures and satisfactions that we can get from living a life: love, education, parenthood, travel, a work life, friendship, and many social activities.

To object that we are all different and have a wide range of values, aims, and hopes about our lives is true. But we are all not *so* different that no generalizations are possible, valid for most people if not for all. Some people, it is true, would like to run marathons at age 90 and do so. But most of us have no such aims, and, in any event, it is hardly self-evident that it is the duty of a health care system to make such ambitions possible or, indeed, that the elderly marathon aspirant at age 90 would have had less than a full life for failing to run because of bad knees. I would like to travel to Nepal, but the absence of such a trip would hardly make my life a failure and less than full because of that omission. Our individual definitions of a full life should not be the norm for national health policy. That is the economically corrosive core of our present system, for Medicare, as well as for the entire system. The health norm should aim, as do all responsible public policies, to find a reasonable way to help us all in a collective manner that takes account of our most common needs and aspirations when it cannot meet all of them. Public policy cannot deliver boutique health care.

In earlier societies, with shorter life expectancies, a "full life" could have been achieved in a shorter period of time, and thus, the length of life and its fullness were not necessarily identical. Do we look back on the deaths of the founding fathers of our country, mainly in their 60s and 70s, as a national tragedy, as if they had died prematurely, their lives incomplete, their lives less than full? No one has ever, so far as I know, said that, and why should they? One can, however, say that it was a tragedy that so many women of that eighteenth century era died in childbirth and that so many of the children of that era did not survive to adulthood.

DRAWING ON EXPERIENCE

I present the notion of a "full life" as a social and experiential concept, based on my own observation and experience of living a long life and of trying to make sense of the different stages of life and the varied reactions to them. In any case, it is open to my readers to compare my observations with those of their own. My suggestion of 80 years as an upper boundary is of course in one sense arbitrary—why not 79 or 81? But for policy purposes, it represents a reasonable number, much the same as the age of 65 was a reasonable number for Medicare eligibility, or 16 for a driver's license, or 21 for drinking alcoholic beverages. I do not mean for that particular age to be used as a rigid standard, much less written into law. I see it instead as a strong signal to patients, families, and physicians to shift gears, raising the bar for aggressive technological interventions, which a use of QALYs will bring about, but also in ways that take account of patient and disease differences.

I first began thinking about the idea of a full life at funerals, noting the great difference in the reaction of those gathered to honor the deceased depending on his or her age at death. I have rarely noticed signs of strong grief and weeping at the funeral of those over 80, and often not even at funerals of those over 70. My mother died at age 86, and those who came to her funeral did not cry but, instead, spoke about how much they liked her, what a fine person she had been, how she had lived a "full" life, and said that she "would be missed." The funerals of young children or adult parents with small children are entirely different (one of our own children died). Grief overcomes most of those who come (and they come in much greater numbers), and it is hard not to cry.

Why is there that difference? I think that it is no accident, and that we know through our experience and observation the difference between someone who had not lived a long and full life, who still had many significant stages of life and experience before them and one who has not. The latter is what we mean by a "premature death." There is, moreover, a difference between a death that is tragic and one that is sad but expected and accepted, and that is the fundamental difference between the death of the young and the old. Another influence on my thinking has been the reading of obituaries for many years, a habit that grows with age, and particularly when one's own age group begins to gradually die off. It is hard to think that someone who has lived into his or her eighth decade, who once pursued and then retired from a career, who had children and grandchildren, had not lived a full life even if there were a few more things that person might have wished to do.

I call my idea of a "full life" a quasiempirical concept; that is, it is based on my observations, its frequent use by others in our society, and because it helps to explain some phenomenon of aging and death that does not seem otherwise explicable. For thinking this way, I have been called a "mortalist" and an "apologist," someone who seems to fatalistically accept aging and death instead of taking full arms against them.[5] I plead guilty to the charge. I cannot imagine running a long-term affordable and sustainable health care system without a citizenry that is willing to accept aging and death, even though with ambivalence and reluctance.

The push by "transhumanists," for a much extended human life expectancy of 150 years and more is no help to our common future and surely a seductive distraction from decent care for the elderly (see chapter 6). The idea that death is just a correctible biological accident and aging a conquerable disease like any other, are the ideas of a small, but growing, minority. But I suspect they have some influence beyond their numbers, attractive to a culture looking for medical miracles and fed a steady diet of hope and hype. A British sociologist has made a good case that utopians who want to carry out a "war" against old age "share a dominant cultural view that devalues old age and old people."[6]

When I was earlier criticized for wanting to use age as a decision-making standard, I often responded with two questions, which hardly anyone took the trouble to answer. If you do not like age to count in determining treatment, does that mean that the elderly are to be entitled to any and all treatments regardless of the cost and that the 9-year-old must compete for life-saving resources against the 90-year-old on a level economic playing field? Or does it mean that an expensive treatment at age 85 that ensures only a few extra months of life should be provided? No one seemed quite prepared to say that; but neither did anyone offer an alternative standard. Questions of that kind make everyone uncomfortable. They put the cost problem to the ultimate test, which is one reason why trying to mix the cost of health care and our commitment to the value of life is acutely discomforting.

I have frequently asked my critics this question: if you think my approach is harsh—even though you agree there is a problem that will get all the worse as the baby boomers retire—tell me what your harsh solution is? No one has ever offered such a solution. They have proffered instead sweet, Alice-in-Wonderland alternatives: more and better medical research to cure the diseases of the elderly, programs to cut waste and inefficiency, dreamy scenarios of modernized life styles for the elderly, and do not believe future cost projections anyway. At least at age 79, no one is likely to ask me, as all did 20 years ago, whether I would still think that way when I was old. Getting rid of questions like that is one of the benefits of old age. To be sure, it could be said that, at 79, I am like most elderly people set in at least a few old-fashioned ways, unable to entertain new possibilities, fresh and transformed ways of thinking about, and living, old age. That may well be true, but it does not alter the fact that my feelings on the subject have only become intensified with age, living with it myself.

RESISTING MARGINAL BENEFITS

One of the afflictions of affluent societies is the unrelenting quest for something more "novel" or "better" than what we now have, whatever it is that we do not have. The economic historian Joel Mokyr has suggested ironically that the slogan, "If it ain't broke, don't fix it," is the greatest obstacle to technological progress.[7] Most new medical technologies do not bring about a dramatic improvement in health but only a slight marginal gain. I have in mind here two senses of marginal benefit. One of them is that of treatments or technologies that provide a low probability of improved health for everyone suffering from a particular disease, one case in twenty for instance, but without knowing in advance which patient will be helped. The other is that of benefiting everyone in a group of candidate patients but to a minor extent only and at a high aggregate cost. Both kinds of marginal benefits can be attractive to doctors and patients. A low probability outcome of either kind for a critically ill patient looks better than a zero outcome if nothing is done. It is not irrational in such cases to want to use the technology: it can just be very expensive and thus harmful to the health care system even if, at times, beneficial to individual patients.

Some recent debates about the implanted defibrillator, an expensive ($50,000) device standing by to deal with a sudden cardiac arrest, have focused on the actual benefits to patients, the subject of increasing doubt. Ninety percent of those who have them (some 140,000) receive no medical benefits and are at risk of various side effects. There is, however, no good way of determining just who is most at risk. In terms of population health, the device is clearly a marginal benefit, but not for those individuals whose life is saved.[8]

The marginal benefit problem is clearly displayed in the gap between high- spending countries and regions and those that spend less. An intensified use of technology is a mark of the former, but it does not correlate with better health outcomes. Nonetheless, there is no slowing of the onslaught of new technologies and intensified use of old ones. Many of these would fail any serious cost–benefit test (at least one using QALYs). Although longer lives are welcomed by most people, it is clear that they do not lead to lower health care costs, and the fact of a small decline in the use of acute care (but not long-term care) medicine by those over 80 may indicate the spread of expensive technologies to a larger number of younger people.[9] The earlier cited study by Dana P. Goldman and his colleagues (see chapter 1), about the poor prospect of many new and expensive technologies lowering costs, is worth recalling here.[10]

The economic necessity of minimizing technologies that promise only marginal individual benefits, and thus, promise little population-wide health benefit, should, I would agree, admit of exceptions. An obvious case would be when the treatment would, if acceptable, promise to restore the patient to an average future life expectancy for his or her age. This exception would favor younger patients, but less likely to have multi-organ failure, and be less favorable to older patients. Low-probability treatment of the elderly in the case of life-threatening conditions should be permitted when the probability of the length of life after the treatment is the same as, or close to, the life expectancy of a person at age 80 prior to the needed treatment. A person, that is, who incurred a lethal disease at age 82 would be eligible for life-saving treatment if there were a good probability that, if cured, or put into long-term remission, the person would live to the normal projected life expectancy of someone aged 80 (e.g., another 7–8 years). The treatment would be discouraged, although not flatly rejected, if the gain in life expectancy would, say, be only an additional 2 to 3 years. A supportive determination would be the QALYs score for the patient. The highest costs are incurred in the last years of life, but they have been the least studied.

CARING FOR THE CRITICALLY ILL

A good deal of research in recent years has shown that it is not age per se (so far) that is responsible for high medical costs but, instead, the remaining time in a person's life before death. That remaining time often comes when there is a hospital-based full court technological press. The last year of life is typically, although not always, the most costly year, and the costs increase in the dwindling months before death, with 51% of these in the last month.[11] Some 26% of Medicare costs are caused by the 5% of the beneficiary population in the last year of their lives.[12] At one time that figure was taken, by some, to indicate a "waste" of money, but it came to be understood (at least by researchers) that this time:cost ratio does not prove the money is being wasted. It only shows that critically ill, terminal patients are usually, as common sense might suggest, more expensive to care for than those who survive, a point as true of younger as of older patients.

It is no coincidence that there is also a strong correlation between the costs of the critically ill and time spent in a hospital. One illuminating study showed an exponential increase in hospital time among those approaching death, some 48% of them being in hospitals for the first time, and nearly 60% dying in a hospital.[13] Yet for those over 80 years, their medical costs prior to death decline in comparison with younger groups, and even more so over age 90. Just why that happens is not clear, and although covert age-rationing might be surmised, it is just as likely that these patients' frail condition and multiorgan failures made them poor candidates for aggressive interventions. In the Medicare studies, those in the last year of life had an average of four major diseases compared with just one for those who survived.[14] Costs for minority patients were 28% higher than for others, suggesting that they arrived at death's door in worse health than nonminorities.

Probably the most telling studies of the critically ill and dying found that some 50% of general health care costs come from some 5% of the population, those who are critically ill.[15] The top 1% incur slightly over

25% of the costs. One-half of the population consumes only 3% of the costs, a figure that has been steady for the past 25 years. The researchers, Mark L. Berk and Alan C. Monheit, commented that

> cost containment efforts were more likely to be effective to the extent that they focused on the very ill. Over the past decades, however, policymakers were clearly focused on strategies that would affect the care received by the larger percent of the population. . . . little effort has been targeted toward those who account for the majority of service use. . . . There are serious limitations to the effectiveness of any cost containment strategies that focus on the 90 percent of the population that collectively accounts for [only] one-third of U.S. health care spending. Accordingly, further efforts to control costs will require difficult choices about the level of care provided to those with the greatest need.[16]

The phase "those with the greatest need" displays a rare willingness to go directly to the most troubling ethical core of serious cost containment efforts. Those with the "greatest needs" are often, by definition, those who will gain the least benefit. And even if critical care costs have historically gone down with the oldest patients, it is hardly self-evident that the same trend will show itself with the coming influx of baby boomers. As other researchers have noted, "one would expect elderly people to demand better and more health care than they used to because of a better financial position and because of changes in attitudes . . . and increased life expectancy [that] may . . . make physicians more likely to use aggressive treatments that were previously withheld for fear of lack of efficacy or harmful side effects."[17] Even apart from acute medical care, the common estimate is that, despite a decline in hospital and acute care interventions, increased life expectancy will not lower elder costs, with increased long-term care keeping lifetime costs high.[18]

REDUCING REGIONAL VARIATIONS

The work of John Wennberg and his associates at the Dartmouth Atlas project decisively shows enormous discrepancies in regional, and even urban, Medicare spending patterns. The differences in the cost per person reflect in part regional variations in general costs but, much more, variation in practice and treatment patterns. Patients in high spending areas "have more visits, hospitalizations, stays in ICUs, and diagnostic tests."[19] No less striking are the variations in available resources, particularly the number of hospital beds and physicians. These variations can be seen among hospitals with high reputations for quality in the same city and among academic medical centers. Patients in New York University Hospital average 76 physician visits per person versus 24 visits at the Mayo Clinic. States that rely on primary care physicians rather than specialists tend to have lower Medicare spending and use fewer ICU beds. The UCLA teaching hospital uses 2.5 more specialists than primary care physicians, whereas the University of California San Francisco medical center uses 1.2 times more primary physicians than medical specialists.

By far the most important finding is that the "the extra spending, resources, physician visits, hospitalizations and diagnostic tests provided in high spending states, regions, and hospitals doesn't buy longer life or better quality of life. In fact, those with chronic illnesses who live in high rate regions have slightly shorter life expectancies and less satisfaction with their care."[20] That statement is backed by a study by the Dartmouth group to determine the health implications of regional differences in medical spending.[21] Their recommendation that the best performing health systems be used as a benchmark is eminently sensible. "The evidence," they say, "that the outcomes and quality of care tend to be better in regions with lower resources shows that providers serving such regions are not rationing care. On the contrary, they are more efficient; they achieve equal and often better outcomes with fewer resources."[22]

They go on to say, in a way supportive of my own population-oriented approach: "The reallocation of resources from the acute care sector to create a population-based, community-wide integrated system for managing severe chronic illness is today only a thought experiment. It should become a national goal." Beyond those domestic studies, however, the evidence is solid that European systems provide considerably less access to medical technology than does the United States but are more popular with their citizens and get a better health outcome for less money.[23]

MEETING UNMET NEEDS

A curious feature about most descriptions of unmet needs in health care is that, with the exception of long-term care for the elderly, those needs fall into the lower categories of my suggested levels of care. They include the unmet needs for hypertension and cholesterol-lowering drugs, for more primary care physicians as well as geriatricians, for more prevention programs focused on behavior change. There have been few complaints about a shortage of ICU or hospital beds, of transplant or cardiac surgeons, or of the latest and best diagnostic screening devices. But there have been complaints by physicians about the helpful movement toward low-cost treatment facilities, such as those being offered by Wal-Mart and other groups. Inexpensive care of minor medical problems, even if not quite as good as mainline care, seems to me a fine tradeoff. In short, there is every reason, in the name of health and cost management to go after the unmet needs, often the less expensive treatments but affecting the largest number of patients.

Eliminating Inequities

There is a rich and important body of research on the inequities in American health care, affecting the poor and minority groups. Because these inequities are borne by various groups as a whole, not just scattered individuals, they are obvious targets for concerted reform efforts. Although many of them bear on expensive treatment needs (such as dialysis and kidney transplants for blacks, and for neonatal ICU care for premature black babies), a large number of them require an improvement at the lower levels of care (immunization of children, screening for diabetes, better access to primary care), which once again indicates the importance of improving the lower levels of medical care rather than the higher. To be sure, many of the inequities reflect poverty and the lack of other social resources, of which poor health is a direct correlation. Much that is necessary to make the lives of the poor better is missing, and that includes health care as well.[24]

HEALTH CARE BY AGE GROUPS

I now want to show that there are two ways of deploying a population health perspective in the care of individual patients, both of which make possible the use of medical necessity as a social, not individual, concept.[25] The first is that of carrying out research, using technology, and allocating resources by the use of age groups as key categories. We do that already with special programs and policies for children and the elderly, and this monitoring could be done with all age groups. The second way is that of prioritizing different levels of health care, but doing so by assessing the relative likelihood of people needing different kinds of care (whether expensive or inexpensive), with the statistically most common needs having the highest priorities.

CHILDHOOD

As a result of medical progress, an improved standard of living, and the sharp drop in morality rates, childhood is now the healthiest stage of life, and the odds of surviving childhood in the United States are now exceedingly good. The death of a child seems particularly tragic in part because it is so uncommon. By and large children are now spared the infectious diseases that killed so many in an earlier time and are not old enough to contract the chronic and degenerative diseases of later life (even if some children still contract cancer, heart disease, and other terminal conditions). Nonetheless, the rise in childhood obesity and asthma in recent years shows that new threats to children as a group can still arise.

Given the generally good health of children, their greatest need is for good and relatively inexpensive preventive medicine, on the one hand, and for a solid family life, on the other. The health care system can provide inoculations, dental care, surveillance for mental health and behavioral problems, and health promotion–disease prevention efforts. The latter should particularly focus on establishing healthy patterns of life (diet and exercise at all stages of childhood and antisubstance-abuse efforts in the adolescent years). A full range of technologies is appropriate. Yet it is evident that the role of parents is crucial for the health of children and not only because parents must be the ones who watch over their children's health. The lives of the parents must be stable and their own health good for them to well discharge that duty, which gives the middle adult years a special societal importance.

When acute care medicine is needed, marginal benefits are most acceptable at this stage of life. Low probability treatments, for instance, should be more tolerable, but never to the point of excessive risk-taking with a child in a way that may severely compromise the rest of her life. And although this strategy will surely benefit individual children, its main purpose is to get children as a group off to a good health start in life for the sake of the future society. Just as good public education has as its principal aim an educated society (the historical reason for the establishment of the public school system), so the aim of child health care is a future healthy society.

Young Adulthood, Ages 18–35

After children, young adults are the next healthiest group in our society. They are a group going through higher education, choosing careers, entering marriage and starting families, but, if they are poor, they are at considerable risk for unemployment and behavior-related health problems. Many young people with moderate income might afford health care but choose to gamble instead and not get it, confident that they will beat the low probability of serious illness. They might get away with that, but they would be better off with health care. Substance abuse, mental health problems, and accidents are their greatest threats, and special priorities should be given to them in the health care system. Beyond that, the childhood emphasis on health promotion and disease prevention should remain strong: the stage is still being set for the more difficult health years to come. If young adults become critically ill, treatments with marginal benefits may be acceptable because they have many potential years left to their lives; and this may be so even if the quality of those lives may be, in the eyes of others, low. A full range of technologies is appropriate, but with the poor, a full range of complementary educational and social services also would be warranted.

Later Adulthood, Ages 36–70

If the emphasis in childhood and early adulthood should remain heavily focused on prevention and oriented primarily to life style and health-related behavior, later adulthood takes on a singular importance. This is the age group that is most responsible for the raising of families and the running of society. The infrastructure of society is their main responsibility, and it has a special need for their good health in a way not quite true of younger age groups.

With the latter groups, it is primarily their future health that is at stake: their present health is on the whole likely to be good. With later adults (ages 55–70), it is their present health that should be the main focus. It is at this stage of life that serious disease and illness begin to make their appearance, and increasingly so as people become older in its later phase. Life-style efforts and behavioral prevention methods remain important, but now the emphasis on diagnostic screening will sharply increase as the probability of undetected but statistically likely pathologies increases. The use of and demand for technology will rise, both for screening and treatment. The once-empty medical cabinets of this group will gradually begin accumulating more vials of pharmaceuticals.

It is here also that the serious dilemmas of technology begin to appear. The social importance of this age group is undeniable. For the welfare of all of us dependent upon them, the standard of medical necessity as a population concept seems most easily met. Research on those diseases most likely to affect this age group is easily defensible. Yet because the curve of the use of technology will sharply rise, the cost of care and the use of technology will rise with it; and they cannot be ignored.

Three considerations are of special importance here. First, diagnostic screening is an area of rapid cost growth. That growth will be a function of patient anxiety and health concerns, of physician training and financial incentives to make use of such screening, and of industry promotional efforts. Screening can be a valuable way to detect illness, and it can also be a great waste of money. The use of QALYs will become more important here, and from a public health benefit perspective, the adoption of moderately stringent criteria for its use seems eminently justifiable. Screening should be undertaken only when there is a comparatively high probability of detecting a pathology and where that probability has been demonstrated. It is here in particular that the popular slogan that "it is better to be safe than sorry" should be most resisted.

Second, in determining appropriate treatments, the emphasis should be placed on procedures that, at the least, promise a good life span prospect and, if not necessarily average life expectancy, then at least enough years for the patient to have come close to living a full life. The marginal-benefit issue can now become especially troublesome, especially when we consider expensive procedures with a low probability of success. It is different with low-cost screening, of which mammography is a good example. The debate about a minimum age for mammography has, for the moment at least, been settled as every two years for those over 40 and every one year after age 50. Given the importance for my revised notion of public health of this age group, some leeway on expensive procedures is probably appropriate, but only if a decent QALYs outcome is possible, and certainly one that might be lower than would be acceptable with the advanced elderly

Third, it is at this stage of life that some long-term, medically manageable, conditions are most likely to put in their appearance. They may reduce life expectancy, but their main impact will be on the quality of life, either because of persistent pain and discomfort (arthritis, multiple sclerosis), a rising number of comorbidities (diabetes), and threats to functioning well in personal and social life (mental health problems, or accident-related injuries). One way or another, these conditions can become, when extended over long periods of time and making use of various technologies (but particularly drugs), cumulatively very costly. A slow decline, often over many years, from a controlled cancer or heart disease is increasingly common. Moreover, these conditions can seriously reduce the possibilities of meeting the conditions of full life, that of experiencing the ordinary pleasures and possibilities of life. Unless the QALYs score indicates prohibitive costs, these patients should be treated. They may not achieve a full life, and the life they have may be of a low quality, but they should be given a chance to make it through life as long as that is possible.

Early Old Age, 71–80

By this stage of life, health problems are beginning to accumulate, some life-threatening but many of them falling into the annoying, mildly burdensome, sometimes painful category. In my own case, that means high blood pressure and a combination of moderate asthma and COPD, enough to cause me breathing problems, eliminating tennis and jogging, and an enlarged prostate gland that causes too-frequent urination. But I consider myself lucky. Some 20% of my college classmates (now in their mid-70s) have died, and many others have crippling and degenerating conditions. Our medicine cabinets have accumulated more drugs, our sex life has declined, our pace has slowed. By current standards we are splendid candidates for diagnostic screening, and even if we are not enthused, our physician or our spouse puts pressure on us that is hard to resist.

Yet by this age, I believe, the baseline standards for both diagnostic and therapeutic procedures should be raised. Although many of us will not have reached age 80, my rough outside boundary line, we will be near it. We may have major unfinished life agendas (though I know few people my age who would say that of themselves), and some of us with no agendas simply want more life, as much as possible. But it cannot be said that we are anywhere near as important for the welfare and vitality of our society, or for the welfare of our families, as when we were younger. Few of us have heavy social or occupational responsibilities, and, although our families would personally miss us, our passing would not much affect society. Those obsessed with antiageism may not like to hear such things said, but I believe them to be true; and one of the realities of old age that takes a bit of getting used to is that fact, like it or not.

We may be sad to read the obituary of an old friend and can certainly feel some special pain when we read of the death of a young person. But despite the fact that most obituary pages these days report the deaths of people over the age of 70, when the majority of people begin to die, I have never heard of anyone who has wept for all those deaths collectively each day or much less said, as Mr. Kurtz did in *The Heart of Darkness*, "oh, the horror, the horror." Nor have I ever heard anyone say, on passing a cemetery: "What a tragedy there are so many dead people there." Part of getting old is knowing that, just as others die, I will also die, but that life will go on.

During this stage of life, diagnostic screening should not be undertaken unless there is a family history of a particular disease, or the screening is for generally health-threatening conditions (high blood pressure and cholesterol levels, colonoscopies) with wide prevalence and low treatment costs. Only high probability threats merit screening, as with mammographies and colonoscopies. As for treatment, the use of QALYs should and will begin to have an increasingly negative effect on the use of expensive medical procedures; they will become economically unjustifiable in a way they were not at the adulthood stages. Some will complain that this makes them ageist in their impact, discriminating against the elderly. But the whole purpose of the use of QALYs is to discriminate (and if it turns out that this aim affects the elderly, so be it), and to do so when we have no other good or fair ways to limit care, and do not wish to invoke the useless standard of individual medical necessity. As for other forms of medical and social support—to relieve pain, to provide rehabilitation, to allow independent living as long as possible, to provide long-term nursing and home care—they should be fully provided. But the emphasis, financially and otherwise, should be shifting to care, not cure, a good quality of life, not a longer life.

LATER OLD AGE, 81+

Historically, those over 80 use far less acute care medicine than those who are younger. Because this has been happening for a long time without any policy efforts to bring it about, is there any reason to worry about costs (other than long-term nursing care) for this age group? Two questions that cannot at this point be answered are (1) whether the baby boomers will bring to their later old age a different attitude toward aggressive high technology medicine than their parents generation, and (2) whether they will go into their old age in worse physical shape as well, a function of growing obesity for example?

There is no way at the moment to answer those questions, but it is reasonable to speculate that, as life expectancy increases, the problems now commonly encountered by people in their 60s and 70s will gradually become pushed into the 80s and 90s (just as the average age of nursing home patients has increased in recent years). The frequent anecdotal reports of physicians about their baby boomer patients, whose demands and expectations for near-miraculous medicine far exceed those of earlier generations and the rising proportion of whom want "everything possible" done to save them at the end of their life, are not reassuring. The rising age of advanced technological procedures noted earlier in the studies of Janet Shim et al. in chapter 2, page 49 already visible, presages staggering future increases.

That possibility means, however, that some kind of preventive cost control steps will need to be taken to dampen that trend. The baby boomers should know that if in their 80s they come to want the same level of technological care they received in their earlier years, they will simply not get it. They need to be put on notice about that, which would be best done by a Medicare policy that makes use of QALYs with well-advertised and steadily rising limits on expensive acute care, and strong resistance to treatments with marginal benefits. Most important, they should understand that the era of endless, open-ended progress and technological innovation with no thought given to costs is over. It will be no less understood that people are expected to age and die, as they have always done, that utopian visions of life extension will not be pursued, that it is not the duty of a health care system to continue the wars against death in old age, or the right of patients to demand it. It is not that utterly different criteria would be used in the care of the old and their access to treatment. Instead, the point would be that, with aging, the criteria used with the elderly would be raised to a higher, more demanding level.

A Policy Dilemma

Although I am particularly thinking about the Medicare program in the discussion of the elderly, a program that would in the future use cost–benefit analysis and QALYs as part of its decision-making on benefits would have to confront a profound policy dilemma. If we set limits on benefits and the use of technology, that would inevitably generate ineq-uities: the affluent could buy, outside of the program, treatments and technologies denied them within it. Yet if we set the standard of cover-age, the basic package, so high that the affluent could, along with every-one else, get whatever it is that they want, we would be back in the present and in the company of a useless individual medical necessity standard; that is, what got us in economic trouble in the first place. Still, if we permit the affluent to buy what they cannot otherwise get through Medicare, then the appearance of inequity will be strong.

There are some possible ways to deal with this problem. One way would be to do what Canada has done, that of outlawing the purchase of private health care (for physicians and hospital care) outside of their national universal care system (though Quebec has declared that policy unconstitutional for that province). The result of that policy has not been a happy one. There are long waiting lists for many forms of care, and many affluent Canadians come to the United States to buy care not otherwise purchasable privately, in Canada. Not only do many Canadians not like that policy, but it has been a favorite debating point for promarket Americans, who see it as a perfect example of the evils of "single payer" and "socialized" medicine. The European coun-tries rarely have such problems, in part because they provide good com-prehensive care, care of a kind that does not ordinarily lure the affluent to other countries or lead to waiting lists but also allows some parallel private care.

Another way to handle the situation would be to encourage people at a younger age to buy insurance for catastrophic care costs. Some might well do so, but the experience of attempting to develop and sell policies for long-term care has not been notably successful because of their cost and the difficulty of persuading the young that they will need such policies; and there have been complaints about the difficulty of gaining money from the insurance companies when it is finally needed as well. It might also be possible to increase co-payments and deductibles at least for the affluent for expensive forms of care. Whether that would produce a significant amount of savings is not clear, which would be a function of their severity. Then we might simply let the inequities exist, and do so on the grounds that the present system, which has no limits, is gradually creating even more inequities through the steady increase of the uninsured, and that, no matter what the system, there will be no feasible way of stopping the affluent from buying whatever they want. If the basic package of health care is generally acceptable in taking care of the statistically most common needs over a lifetime with limits but, basically, economically solid, this unofficial additional "tier" may be politically acceptable. But not everyone will be happy.

SETTING PRIORITIES: LEVELS OF CARE

I have now suggested that looking at the provision of health care in terms of the needs of age groups would make more sense than, as we do now, thinking mainly of health care as directed toward particular diseases and disabilities. Traditional therapeutics would still have an important place in the care of different age groups as most pathologies cut across age groups, even if with different prevalence, but the aim would be to go after the various pathologies with a view primarily of the welfare of whole groups. Cancer care, for instance, would require a different approach for working mothers in their adult years with children still needing care than for an elderly person who no longer has such responsibilities. Treatment would focus not just on the disease but on providing the help and money needed for a mother to deal with her life situation.

Within each of the different age groups, it will be important to have policies reflecting different levels of priorities. As categories, the priorities may be pertinent to each age group, but their order of importance will differ. Below are my suggested levels of health care, in the order of their relative importance for societal health. My criteria for ranking them is the statistical likelihood that any of us will need one or more of them over a lifetime.

All of us, for instance, need clean water, just as all of us are likely at some time in our life to need emergency and primary care. Far fewer of us will need an organ transplant or cardiac bypass surgery. The aim of the priority setting is thus social, not individual, aiming to meet the greatest number of needs for most of us. It will also not necessarily put the "neediest" at the top of the priority list, if by that term we mean those with the most urgent individual need for medical care.

The whole point of the use of age grouping, and priorities of care for each age group, is to have a health care system that would aim to push as much health care as possible down to lower basic and less costly forms of care. The immediate aim would be to reduce acute care at the highest levels, those of cost and technology, and aim as well to discourage the development and improvement of medical technologies at those levels. The long-term goal would be the creation of a sustainable system, one whose annual rate of inflation would be no greater than the growth of the GDP. A considerable part of this would be by the more intensive use of preventive medicine at the lower levels, but prevention-oriented medicine geared toward behavioral and life-style changes, not one enhanced by technological screening methods (which should decline along with many other technologies).

But it should be self-evident that an emphasis on health promotion and disease prevention, which would be the carrot, would have to be accompanied by a stick to catch everyone's attention: that of fewer available medical resources in later life, and fewer expensive technologies with tougher eligibility standards for their use. Successful prevention policies will do no economic good if we continue to find clever technological ways to keep people alive when they finally get sick, which they (we, that is) inevitably will. Another aim of this emphasis will be to minimize the need for directly rationing care. That can best be done by not having technology readily available in the first place. As Wennberg's studies and the European experience shows, more and even better available technology does not commensurately improve health, although it surely raises costs.

Here are my proposed levels of health care, in order of priority, but beginning with a generic category that should always apply, from the beginning to the end of life. I envision with these categories a pyramid model, with caring and public health needs at the wide base and expensive technology at the narrow top.

THE GENERIC CATEGORY: CARING

This level is the most basic, assuming that all of us will get sick at some point, and all of us will come down with some disease or other, and that all of us will suffer at more than one point in our lives some distress, mental or physical. It encompasses the relief of pain, hospice and palliative care for the dying, nursing or home care for the elderly and otherwise frail (together with decent economic support); simple mental health programs for the mildly disturbed; basic and decent home and institutional care for the chronically ill, the disabled, the cognitively impaired, the severely mentally ill, and those powerless to care for themselves. It is difficult to imagine anyone's life, full or not, getting off scot free from one or more of those situations. Caring, then, is basic, the bedrock. Other levels then follow.

- Level 1. Standard public health needs: the provision of nutrition, sanitation, housing, clean air and water, and good programs of occupational health, health promotion and disease prevention, and accident prevention.
- Level 2. Immunization and infection control: the provision of immunization and protection against infectious disease, and available antibiotics and antimicrobials to control infection.
- Level 3. Primary medical care: the provision of emergency medicine and primary care medicine, but limited to routine and relatively inexpensive forms of diagnosis and therapy.
- Level 4. General acute-care medicine: The provision of general forms of advanced medical care of a relatively common kind (e.g., routine surgery, injury rehabilitation, intensive mental health care, less expensive cancer and cardiac therapies).
- Level 5. Advanced, expensive, and statistically less common forms of medical care: the provision of highly advanced, expensive medical care but needed by a minority of the population over a lifetime (e.g., extended stays in hospitals and ICUs, kid-

ney dialysis, left ventricular assist devices for heart failure, and recent biotechnological pharmaceuticals to treat a variety of conditions).[26]

A BASIC PACKAGE OF HEALTH CARE

Whether with the private sector via health insurance or with the public sector via Medicare, it will be useful to make use of: (1) general priorities, such as those just listed (or some equivalent list), (2) age categories (of a kind suggested above), and (3) application of the general priorities differentially within each age group. The "basic package" would ideally consist of stages 1 to 4, on the grounds that all of us have a high probability, indeed the certainty, over a lifetime and at every age of needing treatment at each of those levels. For practical purposes, I believe that the greatest efforts should be to improve levels 1 to 3, which have the broadest effect on our health. Clearly it is likely that children and young adults are less likely to need acute-care medicine and long-term care than older age groups, and that those over age 80 will have less need of preventive care (at least of the technological, diagnostic kind).

Research priorities are a different matter. It is evident that childhood diseases and harmful conditions are on the rise, such as asthma and obesity. I would argue that they should be studied more intensively than, say, cancer, which heavily afflicts older adults. Some $3 billion was spent by the National Institutes of Health for the Human Genome Project, whose goal was to map the human genome. A comparable amount of money could now be spent to study those behavioral conditions that lead to obesity and lack of exercise as well as to study reducing environmental and other threats to health. So too, efforts could be undertaken to increase the number of primary care physicians and geriatricians and to reduce the number of specialists (a point to which I will return in the next chapter). More research on the social and economic determinants of good and bad health would be highly useful as well. In short, there should be a way to develop new treatments and technologies to understanding how health needs are shaped by the kind of society in which we live and the ways in which we choose to live our lives and then to developing the means to promote and use technology appropriately to changing those circumstances. For me, the most appropriate circumstance is that we now live, on average, lives long enough to have a full life. The aim should be to bring everyone up to that standard—no more and no less.

Level 5 seems to me to pose the most difficult problems. They are of three kinds: care for those with statistically less common conditions, but often treatable (and passing QALYs criteria) although highly expensive to do so; care of those suffering from lethal chronic conditions but whose course is slow, expensive, and uncertain; and care during the last year of life, identified as the most expensive and technologically intensive phase of a patient's lifetime. It is here that the problem of medical technology is most acute, with the highest expenses but with much less likelihood of social benefit. It is here also that the idea of "the common good" shows some of its pitfalls.

Uncommon but Treatable Conditions

An obvious objection to my approach would be with patients who have statistically uncommon but far more serious conditions and who can be successfully but expensively treated with the prospect of a good long-term outcome. In my judgment, those patients should be treated. If we can rarely be blamed for our illnesses, we can even less be blamed for contracting statistically rare diseases; but their very rarity will limit their aggregate costs to society.

Caring for the Chronically Ill

An increasing number of patients suffer from conditions known to be ultimately lethal but whose downward slope is of uncertain duration. These patients may be sustained and their life expectancy extended by expensive pharmaceuticals or surgical procedures. If their QALYs score is good, then there is no reason not to provide the needed technology and others forms of care. If those scores are poor but also uncertain, it may still be wise to continue treatment, but less aggressively.

Care during the Last Year of Life

As it often turns out, neither patients nor their doctors may know in advance that a particular time is the last year of life. If a patient in otherwise good health takes a turn for the worse, then it is perfectly appropriate to aggressively treat that patient with a full panoply of technology. If, however, the patient is suffering, as many elderly do, from multiorgan failure with a poor future prognosis (and a poor QALYs score), then it would be appropriate to treat in a less expensive and less aggressive way, testing whether the patient had sufficient resiliency left to survive on his own. In other words, do not give up on the patient, but also do not act as if nothing less than an all-out campaign to save the life is necessary. For a child, that might be just the right thing to do, but not with a patient of advanced age.

Even from a population health perspective, I confess, I am not sure it will be possible to get these three categories quite right. If we go too far in the direction of expensively treating a small minority of patients, or become too lenient with marginal benefit treatments, we will find ourselves right back where we are now. To really control costs, we will have to move in a more stringent direction, and that may be harmful to some individuals. But if that is the price to be paid for a health care system accessible and sustainable over the long term, it may be the only realistic way to go.

CLINICAL DILEMMAS AND PUBLIC POLICY

I will not continue trying to imagine the almost innumerable different scenarios that might present themselves. That course could require a book of its own, and it would be filled with frustration. How can a health care system that needs to control costs be created, much less survive, in a culture that rarely takes "no" for an answer? How can the public be persuaded to reduce its demand for health care in a culture saturated with medical and research boosterism, promising always better health— costly yes, but surely "worth it?" Can a fair system exist in a culture where the gap between rich and poor is widening and where the affluent can readily buy what their health insurance does not provide? And what kind of rationale could be offered those who could not afford to buy themselves out of their health difficulties and would be forced to accept "no," like it or not?

In Britain NICE makes use of QALYs but rejects the use of an absolute threshold for judging the acceptability of a technology in the National Health Service for a number of reasons: "there is no empirical basis for deciding at what level a threshold should be set [but there would have to be 'special reasons for accepting technologies with ratios over €25,000–35,000 as cost effective']; there may be circumstances in which NICE would want to ignore a threshold; to set a threshold would imply that efficiency has absolute priority over other objectives (particularly fairness)."[27] Ethics committees, using some broad and agreed-upon rules and principles are now a common method in hospitals for dealing with difficult ethical dilemmas. But they are rarely called upon to make allocation decisions, much less to tell doctors and patients what they cannot have because a procedure or medication is too costly. They will probably have to begin doing so, however, particularly for dealing with the ethical problems that will arise at level 5 where the complexity with individual patients often does not lend itself to simple principles for making decisions.

Perhaps what I find most frustrating in trying to think through cost control, and particularly technology costs, is that it most probably, almost certainly, cannot be achieved without a government-regulated universal care system. The siren songs of competition from the conservative side, or an incremental improvement in efficiency from the liberal side, should be taken with a grain of salt: they may make a difference here and there, but they have not worked well in the past on any large scale, and they offer no enhanced hope of doing better in the future. Moreover, a universal care system would have to make use of a national budget cap, one that would force everyone and every institution to live within set limits. But that development in turn would not work with technology control unless it was understood that the commitment to technological innovation would (1) have to be seriously dampened, requiring either the voluntary help of industry or the use of financial disincentives that would force it to change in the introduction of new technologies, and (2) much more stringent criteria for the use of old technologies. In sum, the medical technology industry would have to shrink, the use of technologies diminish, the proportion of physician specialists decline and primary care physicians increase. Any other scenario for controlling costs is a fairy tale.

In the final chapter I lay out two possible courses, one that if adopted could work, and one, although still a long shot, would offer a compromise approach to these problems.

CHAPTER 8

GETTING OUT FROM UNDER

The Politics of Pain

Cost control and particularly the management of technology will be painful, necessarily so. It will mean giving up some benefits long taken for granted. It will mean saying no on many occasions to doctors, to patients, to health care administrators, and to industry. It will mean trying to justify what will seem patently unacceptable: your expensive care may be good for you but harmful to the rest of us. It will mean saying that a marginal benefit will not be covered by private insurance or Medicare, while at the same time conceding that "marginal" is not the same as "useless"; it could be even life saving for some patients.

Most people understand that we cannot always have what we want and may need in life. But they are likely to assert about health care, as many have said to me over the years, "that's true enough, but not if it's my wife, mother, or child." Statistics and probabilities are the *lingua franca* of most of us intent on finding ways of controlling costs. They are rarely compelling for sick people. To tell someone that her life might be saved by a new cancer drug, but that it is just too expensive to use, will not be warmly received. Many people, desperately hoping for a cure of a so-far incurable disease, would feel severely cheated to hear that research priorities are to move in a more cost-effective direction. Still others would find that, because of age and multiorgan failure, they or their elderly family members would not be considered economically sound candidates for expensively aggressive efforts to save their lives. Their families would no doubt feel outraged. And politicians will of course be loath to tell the public that stories of that kind are just what the public is in store for if serious cost control is pursued. The outrage will be showered on them.

Access to technology is certain to be the lightning-rod of cost-cutting, more so than reducing physician fees and cutting hospital reimbursements. It will be the most visible and direct sign that spending cuts are being made. Further aggravating this problem, the internet is likely to make the options for care all the better known to patients. Public confidence in the efficacy of technology is high, and habituation to its availability and use endemic. Giving up powerful expectations, even if poorly based in medical reality, is hard enough. Giving them up in the name of such abstract entities as "society," the "common good," or "affordable national health care," is a large stretch, not easy at the bedside of a specific here-and-now person.

Even if we know that, in principle, more technology from a population perspective does not necessarily produce improved health, we also know from an individual perspective that it may help some patients, perhaps save their lives even if it is harmful or useless for others. The desires to live and not to suffer are not only enduring human traits, they are basic ones that have been fed and endlessly stimulated by real medical advances, by excessive hype for those to come, by research promissory notes, and by a public often desperate to reach out for whatever hope it can get, and willing to believe all sorts of unlikely possibilities.

How can we dig ourselves out from the weight of that recent medical history? How can we deal with the burden of excessively high costs, exceedingly high expectations of technological benefits, and an immensely well-financed phalanx of industry and professional groups for whom cutting annual cost growth in half would seem nothing less than a disaster? There are two fundamental difficulties in trying to so, as least from the perspective of shaping health policy. One of them is theoretical, that of fashioning a policy that is coherent, sensitive to many medical and social variables, and whose implications have been thought out. That is what I have tried to lay the groundwork for in earlier chapters. The other, an entirely different kind of enterprise, is to get the scheme accepted in the real world of politics, ideologies, and culture, where the rules and language and fights are vastly different. The need is to close the gap between these two ways of conceiving public policy, each necessary, each different.

I was constantly dismayed in my research to find discussions of the cost problem too often couched in win–win fantasies and hopes. "Higher quality at lower costs" seems to be the most popular example of that, a stitching together of speculative reforms to achieve that aim. Some commentators think it would be regrettable if the health care debate turned into a struggle between improving coverage and reducing costs. Thomas R. Frieden, the New York City Health Commissioner, has written that "if reforming U.S. health care results only in expanded access to care, costs will increase faster but with limited health benefits . . . but [if] only cost controls are instituted, even more individuals will be denied access to needed care. Health care must be structured to make maximizing health the organizing principle."[1] This is in most respects a perceptive comment (but would require universal care along European lines to achieve). Yet the notion of "maximizing health" is in principle a bottomless pit: people will always continue to get sick and die, no matter what the health care system. Maximized health for individuals can only be fitfully and temporarily achieved, to be undone by some inevitable failure of the body; and so it will go until we die.

There is a way of amending Frieden's insight, however, that might be more realistic: health should be maximized in the context of available resources and organization possibilities, and without doing harm to other social and welfare sectors. Reform will be necessary at the organizational level and at the level of our deepest values. A change in our culture will ultimately be necessary to effect reform at both those levels, working to change our addiction to technology and the various economic, social, and professional values that feed and nourish it; and no less to work out a modus vivendi between health care and the medical industry, whose has aims are often at odds with economically viable health care. The political problem will be to find the necessary administrative and legislative leverage to make the requisite changes.

Although I have not in this book come anywhere near trying to lay out a full plan for health reform (nor did I intend to do so), many of my convictions and beliefs have surely come through. Let me sum them up.

- Nothing less than universal care, with strong government oversight and leverage to control costs, will effectively be able to contain cost inflation.
- The European social health systems (SHI) provide better models for the American culture than the tax-based systems (e.g., Canada and the United Kingdom). A SHI system could draw upon the present experience with Medicare, expanding its scope and

combining it with a continuation of employer–employee contributions. That would allow policy to be based on history and experience, a necessity for prudent radical change.

- Although the use of some market practices in health care reform
  might well be effective (e.g., regulated competition among insurers, and freedom of the insured to buy services and amenities
  not covered by universal care), it would be imprudent, even haz-
  ardous, to depend upon unregulated competition to control costs.
  With only a few exceptions, the private sector has not effectively
  and reliably been able to control costs, and the historical efforts
  to foster competition to control costs have at least had a mixed,
  primarily poor, outcome. Deregulation efforts, of which there
  are many, would only make things worse.
- Technology assessment efforts and agencies will have a limited
  impact if they can only make recommendations, if they can only
  commend but not command.

A GLANCE BACKWARD

The aim of cost control should be nothing less than a lowering of the
present annual rate of cost increase down from the present 7% a year
to 3–4% of the U.S. GDP, that is, to have costs grow no more than the
annual growth of the GDP. At the present rate of annual increase, health
care costs in the United States will rise from $2.2 trillion to $4.2 trillion
in a decade. If that happened, the number of uninsured will have increased dramatically, probably to over 55 million, Medicare would be in
shambles, out-of-pocket payments could well be double or triple what
they are now, and even those with good insurance would surely face
severe economic stress, already visible and growing.

How "urgent" is the problem? One meaning of that term is its seriousness, and I believe that the dire cost projections both for Medicare
and other health care costs make that point most emphatically. The other
sense of "urgency" bears on the speed with which this situation must
be addressed. If the cost growth could be cut to 3% next year and continue at that pace for the indefinite future, the projected U.S. annual
health cost in 10 years would be $2.8 trillion, a (more or less) comfort-

THE POLITICS OF PAIN   205

able increase. Under any imaginable scenario, however, such speed is an impossible goal, requiring instant change. We might more hopefully (even if not realistically) imagine a gradual annual decrease over a decade, a rolling average of 5% a year as it moved from 7% to 3%. If so, the annual cost of health care would in a decade be $3.4 trillion.

Are there any reasons to doubt the urgency in both senses? If it takes 10 years to succeed in controlling costs, we will already have pushed the baseline of spending terribly high along the way, and we would have to live with that. The millions of baby boomers are already in the Medicare pipeline, their numbers known and predictable. It is reasonable to expect that they will have higher expectations of medical benefits and more insistent demands than their parents and grandparents. There is increasing evidence that they will go into their retirement years in poorer health than their parents, burdened with obesity and the medical residue of having lived more sedentary lives.

But there are also the contrarians. There are some who believe it does not matter how much we spend on heath care, as good an investment as there is. But it does matter, unless one considers an increase in the uninsured and a decrease in employer-provided care and benefits irrelevant. A few others think the Medicare problem has been exaggerated and that, with modest, incremental changes it can come through. Their thoughts are soothing; but their reasoning is unpersuasive.

The Good News

Faced with what can only be called a stupendous challenge, there is some good news. Although telling rich people they already have enough money rarely works, it is worth noting that, without any more technological innovation at all, Americans will still live longer lives and have better health than any previous generation in our history if, for no other reason, socioeconomic improvement will enhance their health independent of medical care.

In any case, as the European health care systems show, better health can be achieved with far less technology than we are accustomed to. As John Wennberg and his colleagues have also shown, more technology in America does not necessarily improve health, and sometimes can harm it. Additionally, getting rid of regional variation in costs could possibly save 30% of our annual costs. Sarah Brownlee succinctly sums up the persuasive evidence she presents in the title of her book: *Overtreated: Why Too Much Medicine Can Make Us Sicker and Poorer.*[2] And although Robin Hanson may push his point too far, his notion that we could safely cut medical spending in half is worth taking seriously.[3] Estimates that better prevention programs could save us a $1 trillion dollars a year are surely exaggerated, but we could save much. What is theoretically conceivable and what is practically possible are, however, two different issues.

The European example of health care systems that cost less money yet provide better health outcomes and a more satisfied public demonstrate that our way of providing health care is radically defective, and theirs is superior. A Commonwealth Fund study showing that, comparing preventable deaths in the United States with 19 other industrialized countries, the United States comes in last. To make the story even worse, despite our rising costs, far faster then theirs, our progress in lowering preventable deaths is far poorer than theirs.[4] More vexingly, if we had their kind of systems, we would not only be in better shape economically, we would not have to go through the painful transition I projected at the beginning of this chapter for our country to reach an affordable level of care. That hardly counts as good news, but what does is that other countries have shown it can be done.

In December 2007, The Commonwealth Fund released a provocative study showing how a variety of reforms focusing on producing and using better information, promoting health and disease promotion, aligning incentives with quality and efficiency, and correcting price signals in the health care market could, if combined with universal health care, save $1.5 trillion over the next decades.[5] This study is all the more arresting in that it focuses on the possible savings in federal programs only. The savings figures they develop for these different categories were developed by the Lewin Group, a consulting organization whose work is solid and reliable, and they are what it would take to realize the 3% target level for annual cost growth.

I have only two serious reservations with their report. The first, and a point of curiosity as well, is that they did not single out technology as a special problem, as have the Congressional Budget Office, The Henry J. Kaiser Family Foundation, or many health care economists have done in recent years. They leave that problem to the work of a "Center for Medical Effectiveness and Health Care Decision-Making." As I will explain shortly, there are some good reasons not to pin too much hope on such an agency unless it has real clout. My other reservation, also developed more fully below, is that no strategy at all is presented on how their impressive array of cost-savings possibilities could be pushed through politically. Like most studies of cost control, that problem is just not taken up.

THE BAD NEWS AND SOME HARD TRUTHS

The bad news, both practically and symbolically, is the unbroken record of Congress in refusing to allow cost as a consideration in Medicare benefit coverage decisions. Hardly less bad news is the fact that on all three occasions when a technology assessment program was in place, Congress gave in to political pressure, eliminating two of them and greatly weakening a third. The pharmaceutical industry has always successfully lobbied Congress to reject price controls, and the medical industry lobby is one of the strongest in Washington on that and many other self-interested issues. Many (although not all) professional physician associations have rejected interference with the doctor–patient relationship, even when that relationship could help control costs. And everyone loves technology, even when they know in their hearts that it does not always do much good.

Another piece of bad news, rarely discussed, is what might be called the momentum problem. Under the best of scenarios it will take years for even the most effective proposed policies to bear fruit. Short of a presidential declaration of immediate price controls on drugs, devices, hospital charges and those of all medical vendors, and parallel imposed cuts in the fees of medical specialists, nothing else can be done quickly to stop cost inflation. To deal with a broad economic crisis in the early 1970s President Nixon established price controls. They failed and did not last long.

My own judgment is that the health care cost problem is serious enough to warrant such a policy, though it would be difficult to implement. It is no less my judgment, requiring little political insight, that price controls will not be put in place, not now, and possibly not ever. That reality means we are stuck with a range of cost control ideas and proposals that will take years to put into place and at least a decade to bear real fruit. Successful efforts to stem obesity and its medical costs (and other prevention efforts), to establish a national technology information system, to get rid of indefensible regional cost variations, to fully assess new and old technologies, and to radically reduce waste and inefficiency will be slow and will take years. Can anyone doubt that?

In the meantime, costs will continue to rise and, a decade from now, we will have a more expensive system than we now have. The only uncertainty lies in just how much more expensive it will be. If we are as a nation already in trouble with the high economic level of our health care costs, even a slower pace of cost escalation will leave us in a worse state than we are now. Can strong cost controls be all that bad, and sooner rather than later?

There are some hard truths that should never be forgotten in any discussion of cost control. One of them is that we all get old and die, a necessary reminder in the face of "promising" new technologies and cures. We can put off the day of reckoning, but sooner or later our time will run out. Another and related truth is that the cure of one or more diseases in our lifetime, or their remission, opens the way for another disease to take its place, or maybe two, later on. Thus any putative cost savings from the cured diseases will eventually be replaced over our lifetime by the cost of the disease(s) that finally kills us. *Costs need to be reckoned, not medical incident by incident, but longitudinally over a lifetime.* The success of a medicine that can expensively cure a person of cancer at age 65 and of heart disease at 75, only to have that person succumb to Alzheimer's disease at 85, suggests that it is our technological successes, not our failures, that can be the most costly fruits of medical progress.

A final hard truth (or so at least I call it) is the well-documented phenomenon that, as technical progress moves along, it does not necessarily make people happier or more satisfied with life or their health. For an analysis of this phenomenon, see Gregg Easterbrook's book *The Progress Paradox: How Life Gets Better While People Feel Worse*, revealing that medicine is just one more instance of a common modern phenomenon.[6] Dr. Arthur Barsky's illuminating study, *Worried Sick: Our Troubled Quest for Wellness*, found that people now report themselves feeling worse about their health than people 40 years ago did.[7] By every objective test, however, people are in better health now. No doubt this discrepancy reflects a constantly rising baseline of what counts as good health. What we now have is not considered good enough; but, then, it never was and never will be in healthcare. I consider this less-than-reassuring phenomenon the medical equivalent of a dog chasing its own tail, always just out or reach.

THE GREATEST NEEDS FOR COST CONTROL

UNIVERSAL HEALTH CARE

Although I will not number them, I set forth here my version of the greatest needs for cost control in health care in order of priority. I must begin by saying that I did not initially set out when I began this book to present a brief for a universal health care system, but as my research moved along, that kind of system came to seem more and more imperative if health care costs are ever to be controlled. It is not only that the universal care systems of Europe do much better at controlling costs than we do, and with less technology (which is one reason why they do succeed), but that our present public–private mix has demonstrated its incapacity to curtail costs for over 40 years now.

The Medicare program, and the Veterans Administration Health Care System, control costs better than the private sector and could do even better if they were not entangled with that sector. The key to the success of cost control efforts is *control*. The private sector has no organized way of controlling overall health care system costs, nor does it seem to want to do so, and competition among insurers over the decades has utterly failed to stop large annual cost increases. Costs can only effectively be controlled in closed systems that allow overall budgeting, not mixed government—private systems. As individuals, or as corporations, we know we have to live within a budget; no other way of running economically effective private or corporate life makes any sense. What might best be learned from the business community is therefore not competition but the management of budgets.

Yet my judgment that only a universal health care system can effectively control costs must deal with two reality principles. The first is that it is reasonable to project continuing national economic woes for the next few years, and thus the political atmosphere will not be congenial to putting in place a major new entitlement plan (even if it can be argued that a good universal program could hold down cost increases and, in the long run, lead to a more economically sustainable program). The second reality is the persistence of a deep and long-standing ideological gulf in American politics. A Kaiser 2008 election poll asked those surveyed to indicate which of two directions they would like the country to take with health care. Some 43% said they would like to see a policy that built upon present employer insurance with the government paying for the care of those with low incomes. Some 44% said they would like a system in which individuals would buy their own insurance and those with lower incomes would receive a government tax credit to help them pay for the cost of such a plan. In short, a virtual tie. I do not believe that the latter option, obviously dependent upon private insurance, could control costs without a heavy price regulation of premiums.

Jonathan Cohn, the able medical writer for *The New Republic*, is the only analyst I know who worries that universal care, which he supports, could harm technological innovation: "Can we really be sure that universal health care won't come at the expense of innovative medicine?"[8] Once again, the specter is raised of cost controls "stifling innovation." But they probably will and should. Cohn hopes we can have it both ways, contending that much will depend on the kind of system we create: "In fact, it's quite possible that universal coverage could lead to *better* innovation," he writes, and then proceeds to show how that might happen, although he admits it might not happen. Implicit in Cohn's anxiety is the belief that innovation must always go forward, that this progression is a necessary part of medicine. It is surely a valuable part, but then when innovation itself becomes a source of danger for health care, the need arises to rein it in with the recognition that more medical technology does not automatically do us all that good anyway, at least proportionate to its costs. Cohn makes it seem that distinguishing between good and bad technologies is not difficult to do, which it is. Our goal should be, he says, is "to reduce our spending moderately and carefully; the savings, most likely, would materialize over time." Yet none of the previous efforts over nearly 40 years to do precisely that have come anywhere near success. The belief in such comforting outcomes is what got us in trouble in the first place.

LEVERAGE

By cost control, I mean possessing and using the leverage necessary to achieve this outcome. At least fifty ideas on how to control health care costs have been put forth, and I learned much from all of them. But strikingly absent is a political account, even if a somewhat fanciful one, of how these varied plans could be brought to pass; that is, what kind of leverage and clout would take us from "good ideas" to "workable policies?" A well-regulated universal care system could help us do that.

There is no way now that, say, Dr. Wennberg's call for using those cities or regions with the lowest costs as a baseline for all others can be effectuated without the leverage necessary to cross regional and state boundaries and to interfere with the private practice of medicine in hospitals and doctors' offices. Even Medicare has found that hard to do, if only because of great variations in the private sector that effect its operation. Only when states, regions, and cities are forced to toe a cost line, by financial or other penalties, will that be possible.

LEVERAGE AND TECHNOLOGY ASSESSMENT

Despite the failure of earlier government-run technology assessment agencies to survive political and medical opposition, one more try is necessary, and this is a popular idea once again. This time, however, the attempt must be different. The safest and most tempting route, designed to minimize opposition, is that of an agency that only collects data on medical and health outcomes and makes recommendations on best practices, commending and not commanding. That will not be enough. For one thing, the demise of agencies that followed that soft line shows that their softness was not sufficient to keep them alive, and might not do so again. For another, even good recommendations can take years to be developed and even more years to take effect; it is a long and slow process. In the meantime, costs will continue to rise.

The only fully useful technology assessment agency would be one that, like the British National Institute for Clinical Excellence (NICE), has the power to make its recommendations take effect. Technically, NICE only makes recommendations to the National Health Service, but it is understood that, in most cases, they will be followed; only sharp political outcries (which do happen from time to time) can derail them. That is the only kind of agency, I believe, worth aiming for.

NATIONAL PRIORITIES FOR RESEARCH
AND HEALTH CARE DELIVERY

Although the National Institutes of Health is periodically pressed by Congress to explain how it sets its research priorities, it has only rarely been criticized in any major way for what it does; various disease advocacy groups have complained at times about their share of research money.[9] From time to time I have raised with scientists the possibility of organizing priorities in the direction of treatments that would not be costly, but none know of any assured way of doing this, and for a good reason: the NIH essentially does basic research, and there is rarely any way at that level to know what the clinical applications might be, not to mention what their economic impact could turn out to be. There have, however, been persistent complaints that NIH has not invested enough money in health promotion and disease prevention. Because bad health is frequently the result of unhealthy behavior, environmental and social conditions, certainly more money could usefully be spent in examining those factors. The long-time de facto priority given to lethal diseases at the NIH (cancer, heart disease, stroke) is overdue for a reconsideration. Dr. Steven H. Woolf has made a strong case "that the United States should focus as many or more resources on restoring quality as on biomedical advances."[10] His is a lonely but wise voice.

The leading priority should be to push as much health care as possible down to the more basic medical and public health levels and reduce money at the higher technology, expensive levels. The statistical likelihood of a person needing a particular kind of health care at different stages of life should be the standard for setting priorities. The advent in recent years of efforts by Wal-Mart and other organizations to provide inexpensive care in a retail-intensive way is a welcome development. Much more useful health care can be provided by nurses and physician assistants and that practice should be encouraged; efforts will be needed to increase their number. The use of generic drugs can be further facilitated and all the more now that the pharmaceutical industry seems to be running dry of new drugs.

With the exception of a few cost-control ideas—more information technology, formation of a technology assessment agency, and a reduction of fee-for-service medical care—I could find few systematic efforts to sort out the comparatively more and less-promising ways to do so. The Commonwealth Fund study cited above simply presents their wide range of control ideas as a kind of smorgasbord. Just as it does not deal with the leverage need in any clear way, it also does not try to say which of the items on its menu are likely to be the hardest or easiest to digest in a cost-cutting menu.

Because its menu focuses on what the federal government could do, it is no less important to take seriously the organizational difficulty of simultaneously pushing for a wide range of ideas that will involve many federal agencies and step on many toes along the way. Some of the Commonwealth Funds reform directions could probably be achieved within Medicare's existing administrative framework. Others will require congressional action, altogether an enormous political undertaking as well as a considerable bureaucratic task. Which of its ideas are more or less necessary and feasible? A game plan is needed, but it is hard to imagine that anything less than some kind of strong central authority, with full congressional support, could devise and oversee a strong, binding plan.

RESOLVING SIX DILEMMAS

Throughout the preceding chapters of this book, I wrestled with a number of dilemmas, both explicitly and implicitly. Resolving these in some acceptable way, both theoretically and practically, seems. Some of them bear directly or predominantly on Medicare, others on health care more generally.

Dilemma 1: *The need for improved Medicare and other elderly coverage versus the need to slow cost increases.*

Despite the provision of pharmaceutical coverage for the elderly, Medicare suffers from many shortcomings, the relief of which would increase its annual cost: the need for reduction of out-of-pocket expenditures, now becoming prohibitive and particularly painful to former low- and middle-income recipients living on small pensions, social security, and little savings; better coordinated care, particularly for the chronically ill; assurance of the availability of primary care physicians (and an increase of geriatricians); and greater social and other forms of support for independent living for the elderly. Costs that are not directly medical but that have important health implications need to be woven into an integrated program (e.g., long-term care taken out of Medicaid and put into Medicare; social service support for an elderly person trying to care for a sick spouse).

Dilemma Resolution: Any resolution for these problems should involve greater support at the lower levels of basic medical, economic, and social care with corresponding reduction of support for the most expensive hospital and critical care medicine. This mode of resolution embodies a premise I proposed earlier in the book: a health care system should help young people to become old, but not to help the old to become even older; hence, a change in priorities for the old.

Dilemma 2: *Needed technological innovation versus the need to control the introduction and diffusion of new technologies.*
The persistent fear that cost controls will stifle technological innovation rarely considers the question whether any and all innovations are equally necessary—which is whatever the private sector decides to produce—or whether they need be the most important source of future health, as now seems to be the common belief.

Dilemma Resolution: We must shift to the use of a priority system for research and allocation decisions. It should give priority to newly emergent medical needs and to pressing unmet medical needs, but should at same time make coverage for new and improved drugs and devices harder to obtain. Many in the past provided marginal benefits only. Most important is the need to make clear to industry the need to take seriously federal priority guidelines, an important aim of which would be to stifle not all innovation but only that kind primarily concerned with creating new markets, medicalizing life problems, and creating public fears and anxieties to enhance technology profit. Moreover, present knowledge of the social and economic conditions necessary for good population health should make it evident that technological innovation is only one way to improve health. It just happens to be the way most profitable to industry and no less probably the most attractive to the public.

Dilemma 3: *A government-dominated health care system versus a market-dominated, private-sector-oriented system.*

For a number of decades, and from previous reform efforts, it has been evident that ideological differences about the role of the government have been the principal roadblocks to reform; and they are especially strong now. Without some compromises, reform of any significant kind will remain unattainable.

Dilemma Resolution: Note that I use the word "dominated" in both cases, leaving room for each system to make a secondary use of some of the values and practices of the other (as the Dutch are attempting to do by using competition within, and not against, its commitment to universal care). But that kind of nod toward the market and the private sector is a nod only. The private sector in health care has never demonstrated anywhere that it can effectively control national system costs, even if it might do so with parts of a system. When the market functions as a true market, it consists of independent actors, each aiming to maximize its individual profit, not the system's well-being.

Each of the private sector actors has in health care a fundamental conflict of interest. Industry must try to serve health care needs while at the same time satisfying shareholders, whose aim typically is profit, not improved health. Despite all the traditional scorn for the bureaucracy of government, the Medicare program has considerably lower administrative costs than private insurers. Government does not have an inherent conflict of interest and is thus a better vehicle for health care than is the private sector. In the end, government must answer to the public, forcing an accountability that is absent in private sector medicine. Nonetheless, in the name of some kind of détente, I propose two suggestions. If market advocates would concede the need for some government oversight and strong regulation of the private sector in the context of cost control, that would be an important concession. If universal care adherents would admit some market practices (although not unregulated competition) within the context of universal care, that could also be a helpful move.

Dilemma 4: *Individual patient self-definition and physician judgment versus the need for patient care standards based on a mix of public health norms and individual needs.*

By no means all but a significant portion of medical practitioners and some professional organizations have asserted the primacy of the doctor–patient relationship as a reason to oppose strong government-imposed, cost-control measures. There is probably little doubt that this deep medical tradition meets with patient acceptance, reassuring patients that their physician has only their individual health needs at heart.

Dilemma Resolution: The traditional doctor–patient relationship, one of the core values of medicine, can be an obstacle to good health policy, invoked all too often by many physicians to justify practices at odds with the control of costs. It is frequently used to resist evidence-based clinical guidelines, to resist allowing cost considerations to be used with individual patients, and to oppose universal health care in the name of physician freedom. The heart of the objection is to the invocation of scientific probabilities as a guide to patient care: every patient is different, the argument goes, and no one but a patient's doctor is in a position to judge what the appropriate treatment should be; and that the doctor ought to be exclusively interested in my personal benefit. Cost is an alien consideration within that context.

It is not easy to reject that line of thought. It has served us well over the centuries and reinforced trust in the doctor–patient relationship. In one of a long line of physician broadsides against EBM, "Evidence-Based Medicine vs. Patients," Dr. Richard Dolinar of the Heartland Institute has written that because he has the ultimate responsibility for patients, "he should have the ultimate discretion."[11] It is now necessary to qualify that ethic, but to do so only in the name of the health of health care. Regulations and guidelines in the care of patients are needed based on the best science. If each patient is different, as that ethic often insists, then medicine would be nothing more than a throw of the dice with each patient. But medicine has done better than that. It has been willing, through science, to understand that there are some important regularities in patient illnesses; each patient is not utterly different. The art and science of medicine must each receive its due. That balance means that solid evidence must at times be allowed to trump a doctor's professional judgment.

Dilemma 5: *The embrace of a model of medicine that stresses endless and open-ended progress and innovation regardless of cost versus one that is limited in its aspirations and gives priority within a context of finite resources to a good, but not necessarily ideal, quality of life.*

Dilemma Resolution: There is a need for a public and professional recognition of the finiteness of life and resources. That would mean a different set of underlying values about health, aging, and death—a truce with them in place of the present and increasingly expensive warfare against them. There is no obvious or historically instructive way to change deeply held and cherished values, but nothing less is now required for health care. We did that with feminism, the civil rights movement, and environmentalism. It was a long and slow incubation in each case and one heavily dependent upon fortuitous external events to make the historical moment right for change (and many still resist some of those developments).

We have almost, but not quite, reached the right moment for great change. That moment will require another insight, one that most organization-minded reformers resist: in the end there is no good way to manage infinite health desires to overcome aging, sickness, and death with finite budgets; nor is there a good way to pay for a kind of medicine that has chosen technology, whatever its cost, as it principal weapon in an unending, and ultimately unwinnable, war.

Education and sustained public dialogue are the only available lines of defense in resisting the excesses of that war. We must, I believe, stifle the notion of "stifling technological innovation." Unrestrained and cost-insensitive innovation *needs* to be stifled. In its place must be put a prudent, priority-oriented, vision based on prevention, primary care medicine, and low-cost technologies. And that will be more like a guerilla struggle, one aiming to win over populations to effect a truce rather than a heavy-weapon technological blitzkrieg.

Dilemma 6: *Meeting the needs of a growing number of elderly and the rise of Medicare costs versus the needs of younger age groups, particularly children.*

The growing disparity of resources going to the elderly relative to children is not a good development. Children represent the future of a society and thus as significant a share of resources as the elderly, and it is the welfare of children that is now falling behind.

Dilemma Resolution: The rising and expected even greater rise in Medicare costs bring the issue of intergenerational equity, little discussed of late, back in the foreground. I first became interested in this problem back in the mid-1980s, stimulated by a 1984 presidential address by the demographer Samuel Preston to the Population Association of

America.[12] Preston noted a gradual shifting of resources from the young to the old and found that disturbing: "Let's be clear," he wrote, "that the transfers from the working age population to the elderly are also transfers away from children, since the working ages bear far more responsibility for child rearing than do the elderly." That problem has not disappeared; it is getting worse. A 2007 study by the Urban Institute of 100 federal programs found that children's share of domestic spending and tax breaks has declined from 20.1% in 1960 to 15.4% now. Surely some of that shift is due to the increasing number of elderly but also to effective lobbying for their interests. Since 1998, the AARP has spent $105 million lobbying for the elderly, while the Children's Defense Fund has spent $1.3 million.

There was considerable resistance to data of that kind when I first stumbled across it, and it does not receive much attention now. One objection was highly individualistic in its character: all children and all old people are individuals and each has an equal claim to resources. Another was that we all have different needs at different stages of life and that the different generations are not in competition with each other. Still others invoked the necessity (and likely triumph) of research to rid ourselves of the diseases of old age. The idea that we might use age-based rationing to level the playing field was rejected out of hand from all quarters. I was beaten but not bowed for arguing that position which, as will have been noticed earlier, I have modified but not entirely abandoned.[13]

I believe the only reasonable approaches are to concede the greater importance of children and younger age groups for the future than for the elderly and to make certain the economic imbalance does not increase. I would hope the elderly would take the lead in making that case, lobbying Congress and their state legislators for good health and education programs for the younger generation, serving on school boards, and watching out for the welfare of children. Children and young people still have a long life ahead of them and we, the elderly, do not. That last observation is true, and ought to make a difference in how we set societal priorities. Does it make any sense that we spend 16% of our GDP on health care, for a relatively healthy society, but only 5% on education, weak by international standards; yet the former keeps rising, and the latter remains static. Where does the future lie?

POLITICAL STRATEGIES

Ideas for controlling costs are plentiful, and some (as with the Common-wealth Fund study) even have some numbers attached to them. But the plenitude of reform ideas is matched by the dearth of political strategies to achieve them. Simply put, how do we get there from here? My esti-mation, and it is no more than a rough intuition, is that cost control needs to have its own advocacy groups and agendas. They are many organizations and groups pushing for health care reform, on the right for market practices and on the left for universal care, and there are a number of individuals, academic and otherwise, who write about the topic. But as a general rule, cost control is treated as a branch of overall health care reform. It is not seen as a specific topic that should incite the creation of advocacy groups with carefully developed agendas and well-honed techniques for reaching legislators, the media, and the public. But that is just what is needed. The politics of cost control is likely to be far more difficult and complex than simply pressing for coverage of the uninsured.

Cost control seems to be a topic that belongs to everyone in general and no one in particular. If I am correct in thinking that it is a much less friendly topic than, say, the uninsured because of the high cultural place given technology in our society and medicine, then it will be much harder to invoke the kind of passion that inequities do. It is easy to imagine organizing and fighting to help those in need of care, and that is constantly being done, but it is much harder to imagine organizing potent groups that will passionately fight to reduce the influence and excessive use of technology. The latter would, at least in the eyes of many, take something away from people they prize and think they need (and sometimes they will), and not give them anything immediate in return. Nonetheless, that is just the kind of drive that needs to be mounted.

Let me, then, imagine how an advocacy campaign might be organized. Three first steps would be necessary: (1) to formulate the case for cost control, with a particular focus on technology, and with carefully devel-oped goals; (2) to identify a constituency for advocacy, seeking as broad a coalition as possible; and (3) to work to persuade the multiple interest groups with a stake in technological innovation and diffusion, to work together to deal with a problem that effects everyone.

Formulating the Case for Cost Control

The formulation of a case for cost control should not be difficult—on paper. Uncontrolled costs are now everyone's problem. If not better managed, then these runaway costs will it not necessarily destroy our health care immediately (the affluent will always find a way), but they will do lasting damage, create enormous disparities in care, epidemic anxieties about personal health costs, and cause the downfall of many necessary institutions, especially hospitals and even our Medicare and Medicaid programs.

I used the phrase "on paper," because listing dangers and evils do not constitute an effective strategy, especially when dealing with "beloved beasts." What would be an emotionally effective case? The visible deterioration of our present system, spreading economic pain more and more widely, is beginning to make a difference in that direction. The pain can be seen and can be felt. Many of those who have studied the cost problem, amply cited in this book, believe that we can have better health outcomes and a more responsive, efficient system with less technology and lower costs. We know it can be done because other countries have done it; and their experience and outcomes should be readily used to help make the case. In one sense, in terms of our cultural habits and expectations, what needs doing will at first feel painful, but in the long run, we will feel better, our main medical needs will be met, and our financial anxieties reduced. As a distinguished physician friend, Eric Cassell, once said to me, "We take sick people and often make them even sicker in order to make them well." That observation could apply to sick health care systems as well.

False hopes should not be instilled. Real hope can be engendered and supported with evidence, even though the early steps in getting there may be difficult. We will all breathe easier with an annual cost inflation rate of 3% than one that is 7%. We will also gasp for breath along the way.

Identifying a Constituency for Advocacy

A broad-based coalition will be necessary, drawn from every segment of American health care: physicians, nurses, hospital administrators, research scientists, health policy experts, state and federal legislators and administrators, and various public groups. Putting such a group together will mean, however, that it must be drawn from many of the very groups that benefit from high costs and expensive technologies. They will in effect be biting the hand that feeds them. I believe such people can be identified and recruited.

Persuading the Assorted Interest and Ideological Groups to Sit Down Together

If a potent advocacy group could be put together, it would almost certainly provoke a sharp and negative response. It would threaten many interests in a most direct and visceral way. Making use of an experienced and respected negotiator, the advocacy group could attempt in part to preempt some of that likely reaction by bringing the parties most likely to be aggrieved together, to control the tone of the debate, to sharpen the issues, to see where compromise might be possible, and to understand the lethal effects of not solving the problem or putting us on the way to a solution.

In an era of highly charged, often nasty, partisan politics, everything possible to keep that poison out of the room would have to be done. It already seems apparent that the large number of uninsured has not inspired many conservative politicians to be willing to take strong steps to do something about this problem. They want reform but focused at best on reducing the number of uninsured and promoting various market ideas to do so; and the market they believe can, if given a chance, deal with the cost problem. Whether the specter of rapidly rising costs will bring out a more melioristic, ecumenical spirit remains to be seen.

SOME IMMEDIATE STEPS

A number of foundations and research institutes have been responsible for calling attention to the cost problems, mainly by developing ideas to deal with them and generating information and data to show their importance. They would do well now to sponsor some political studies to devise ways to deal with the cost problems and perhaps to seed some advocacy groups as well. They could also bring together various groups and individuals, preferably informally to get a dialogue going and, if progress could be made at that level, the meetings and discussions could be taken to the public. My own experience over the years with many controversial topics is that the talk goes much better, in a friendlier and less grandstanding way, if it begins in private.

If not handled properly, cost control is a topic that can bring out the worst in everyone and is an especially fertile territory for ad hominem attacks. Any mention of cutting back expensive care for the elderly will invite the charge of ageism; and any mention of reducing the use of expensive life-saving technologies for the elderly will add to that charge social euthanasia or murder. To propose that physicians should not always have the final say in the treatment of their patients, or that patients could be denied care of potential benefit to them, will be seen as an attack on physician authority, patient autonomy, and on the doctor–patient relationship. To contend that costs can only be controlled by an organized government response will invite the label of "socialized medicine," a well-known menace.

It is also important to return again and again in any American effort at public and professional education to the European experience with universal care and technology control. The European model is too little known in this country where we have focused attention on the alternative Canadian and British health care plans, which I consider the weakest kind. We have not focused at all on borrowing policies from the continent that could well work here. A foundation that brought some European health care leaders here and took them on a national tour around the country, with ample media coverage, would perform a valuable service. They know things we do not know about cost control and that everyone in this country should know.

TWO REFORM TRACKS: OPTIMAL AND CONCILIATORY

Optimal

By an optimal track I mean one that aims to reduce the annual rate of health care cost inflation to between 3% and 4% and to do so in the fastest way possible. I call this optimal because, based on what we know of cost control methods in other countries, it is technically possible; that is, a health care system as good and probably better than our present one can be run at a lower cost and with a smaller annual cost increase than the present United States system. But "technically possible" does not mean politically or culturally possible. That is the rub.

Even if there is a will to move in an optimal way, the pain and difficulty of doing so will invite evasion, lethargy, foot-dragging, and visible distaste. New contrarians will appear with happier, less painful ideas. The media will quickly pick up on stories of patients denied care, of physicians angry with government interference, and of hospitals forced to close. Legislatures would try to impose mandated treatments, courts would be flooded with legal challenges, and physicians might even strike. Our culture will work overtime against a denial of technology, as will the pharmaceutical, biotechnology and medical device industries, with all their considerable power in Congress to protect their interests.

Worst of all, I would imagine, the denial and the pain would be much more visible and emotionally potent than the benefits. The benefits would only show up over a long period of time, primarily in statistics: death rates would not increase, life expectancies would continue to gain, death rates from lethal diseases would continue to decline. In short, our system would not be hurt, and even be improved by a reduction in the use of technology, but those statistics would not jump out at the casual observer, who might well recall only the individual pain.

It will take uncommon political leadership—not present now—to push an optimal agenda and to concede that, along the way it would entail considerable upheaval and rebellion and many aggrieved patients. But if an optimal plan with all of its political drawbacks is not at least recognized as an ideal, with means and ends spelled out, then it is hard to see how any serious change can ever take place. Compromise will almost surely be needed, but it will work most effectively if shadowed by an ideal to strive for—better that then starting with a compromise and then compromising further.

I will not offer more than a series of bullets with my optimal plan. All of these have been touched on earlier in the book.

- Universal care along the lines of the European Social Health Insurance programs: employer–employee contributions with government support for the poor and aged; the use of government-regulated competitive private insurers; tight controls on the adoption and placement of expensive technologies. The universal care program would have the power to establish national budgets, to control prices, and will make use of a federal cost control agency.

- Establishment of a permanent federal cost control agency in the executive branch, to include the following features: the director of the agency would have the power to make binding cost control decisions, assisted by a national advisory council; and that agency would make use of the findings of a technology assessment agency, which in turn would have the power to make binding recommendations, but which could, under specified circumstances, be overridden. The agency would manage the introduction, diffusion, and use of new technologies and close supervision of older ones.

- The major medical industries that develop and sell new and old drugs, devices, and products would, prior to their release, have to prepare a cost–benefit analysis of them, laying out the health and economic benefits and no less laying out the expected economic impact; and, with already-existing products, they would have to do the same after a five-year delay to allow them to develop a comparable assessment.

- Medical education would be subsidized in order that students can graduate with few or no debts, and those going into the most basic fields of primary care, family medicine, geriatrics, and public health would receive financial incentives for making those choices.

- Physicians would be paid either as salaried employees of medical groups or on the basis of time spent with patients rather than for the use of technological procedures. Subspecialists whose education may have been longer and whose skills are more difficult to achieve should receive no more than a 10% premium for their time. Economic incentives for good performance would be routine.

- The government would subsidize neighborhood clinics specializing in basic ambulatory health care and which in nonemergency situations would serve to screen for emergency or hospital care.

CONCILIATORY

No health reform plan of any substance is likely to be enacted in this country unless it is a hybrid, a mixture of government and private sector features. The persistent public opinion finding that most people would like universal care, but sharply disagree on the form it should take, is not likely to change in the near term; cost control will likely elicit a similar reaction. Although they both agree that technology is a good thing and innovation is to be cherished, liberals and conservatives bring different, if often overlapping, values to their embrace of it. For liberals, technology represents the virtues of scientific progress and human advancement, the most prized intellectual underpinning for human freedom. For conservatives, it demonstrates the good that can come from unhampered scientific research using the power of the market to deliver technology developments with great social benefit.

When it comes to devising a reform health care plan, conservatives might well accept a voucher plan, with government and/or employer vouchers with unregulated private insurers offering competitive choices. Liberals might be willing to accept a Dutch model, with competitive insurers, but only if employed within the context of universal care and with the competition regulated to keep costs under control. Conservatives will be reluctant to regulate technology if choice and competition about its use are hampered. Liberals might tolerate regulation if carried out in the name of equitable care—but I say "might" because many liberals in my experience look upon the regulation of science and technological innovation as a hazard to human liberty as well and are as reluctant to talk about rationing and limits as are market conservatives. They have traditionally wanted both universal care and steady medical progress, and with a focus on individual welfare. They are not comfortable with the language of tragic choices, foreign to Enlightenment optimism.

In devising a conciliatory track, I have tilted it toward regulation of costs, if only because that represents the only reliable and tested method for controlling them, even if that method is more accepted in Europe than here. I will, however, be looking for a plausible balance, but one that would make a difference, even if not enough of a difference to reach optimality. Much will depend on whether costs are seen as a problem, a *serious* problem, an *urgent* problem, or an *immediately urgent* one.

These problems are now being written and talked about, but the degree of perceived urgency is not yet clear. The fact that even the presidential candidates have tended to evade it or to offer weak cures, suggests that the importance and depth of the problem have not sunk in. Or, as an alternative possibility, they have sunk in all to well, and everyone is nervous or terrorized about taking the mammoth issue on. And well they might be if they must deliver, without euphemisms, a message of short-term pain and long-term gains.

- Universal health care may be based on voucher models but give unregulated competition a time trial only: if after a specified time (3–5 years), competition is not controlling costs, then government will regulate insurance premiums and drug prices.
- If universal care is not adopted, Medicare will require costs to be a consideration in benefit decisions, making use of cost–benefit analysis, QALYs, and other economic techniques
- Establishment of a cost control office in the Executive branch, with a designated, prominent, and visible director will be a necessity. Although the director will not be able to do more than commend rather than command cost control strategies, the office should have enough prestige and prominence that the media, medical institutions, physicians, and industries would have to take it seriously. If at all successful, the cost control effort would put everyone on the defensive, forced by public pressure to take seriously its recommendations and be required to give public reasons for dissent. The office should, at its outset, be given a long life, at least 10 years, so that controversial decisions, or ones that offended various interests, could not lead to its elimination or neutering, as has happened with similar past efforts.
- Establishment of a technology assessment agency would be required as a central part of the cost-control agency. This agency would be empowered to develop and collect data on medical technology, to develop experimental and model programs. It would have a variety of powers: to recommend the acceptance or rejection of new technologies as well as those well established. Its recommendations would not be binding, but they would be well publicized and seek to affect public and professional opinion.

- The use of economic impact statements by industry would be required. The technology agency would also have the power to request from the medical industry cost–benefit and other economic evidence of potential health and economic impact of the new and old technologies, and to do so with the new ones prior to their public marketing. Their internal marketing and profit projections would serve that purpose. The cost control agency and the technology assessment agency would then inform the industries about their favorable or unfavorable recommendations for federal and private adoption in response to the information provided. The industry would, however, not be bound by the recommendations but would, if the procedure were transparent enough, be subject to public and legislative scrutiny and criticism if it went forward anyway.
- Special medical education subsidies (or debt forgiveness) would be available for those students pledged to go into primary care or family medicine, geriatrics, emergency and rehabilitation medicine; and additional help would be provided during residency years.
- Financial help and other incentives would be established for clinics and other low-level medical needs (with Wal-Mart or similar efforts as models), to create in effect neighborhood clinics with the manpower necessary to provide good care.
- Tax benefits for corporations initiating health maintenance and prevention programs for employees would be provided, with added incentives if they added compulsory features and financial penalties for employees who fail to comply.
- The bias of government research would be toward low-cost treatments and technologies and disease prevention (and a $3 billion health behavior project).
- A better balance would be sought in Medicare between cure-oriented or otherwise expensive treatments and financial and social support services and better long-term and home care assistance for the elderly. Long-term care would be moved out of Medicaid and put into the Medicare program as part of an effort to integrate all forms of elder care under one umbrella. Recognition would be made as well that the financial situation of elderly

has important health effects and should thus be part of a general package of elder care.

- Although an annual limit on Medicare expenditures would most likely not be politically acceptable, the cost control agency mentioned earlier could put together an oversight group that would issue an annual report on cost-saving efforts, including progress being achieved toward the ideal goal of a 3–4% cost increase per annum that would issue an annual report on progress toward that goal.
- During the transition of putting into place a conciliatory, compromise policy, the public should be made aware of the distance between those current policies and long-term goals, emphasizing always the financial disaster for everyone if the long-term goals are not successfully pursued.
- Continuation and intensification of the Quality Improvement movement; intensification of efforts to develop shared decision making between informed patients and physicians; more disease management programs; reduction of medical error and inappropriate care would all be aggressively pursued.

In writing this book, I wished that I could find some hopeful, inspiring ideas and information to pass along. I did discover some, as noted, but they do not add up to the fast and furious momentum needed to control costs and technology in American health care that seems to me imperative. They often of necessity go against the grain. To speak of some "necessary pain" is not the way to success in politics, save, perhaps, in wartime. To suggest that our beloved technology is not all that good for us is a story that many doctors, all of industry, and most of the public do not want to hear. To say that it is time to stop our health care tradition of slow-paced incrementalism—regularly spiced up with a large dollop of muddling through—and to move on to a full health care reform is to invite scoffing from political realists.

There are realists, however, and there are realists. My way of realism has been to lay out all the reasons that cost control is necessary, to note all the obstacles that stand in the way, to say what I think needs to be done—and finally, to say that it can be done if we are willing to put up with the pain. For if the other kind of realists once again come to dominate the health care debate, we are all in trouble.

CODA

E very author should be allowed at least once in a book to nakedly display his feelings, usually hidden beneath the veneer of scholarly distance and hints of gravitas. He should be allowed at least one tantrum, one fit of confused hysteria, one instance of teeth-gnashing, one outburst of political exasperation, and in this case more than one bout of moral anguish.

My tantrum first came one day when I realized that there are many of my fellow citizens, and even a few health care professionals, who seem unwilling to accept any stance toward cost control that does not deliver a happy outcome. In an updated version of the "the power of positive thinking," they seen to think that optimism and organizational cleverness can save the day. Incremental tinkering will do the job. It is an old American trait, eschewing negativity and dark thoughts.

My hysteria is the result of trying to make sense of a basic tension in what I was reading. On the one hand, there are all the fine and plausible ideas advanced in recent years for managing costs and especially technology costs. They are almost more than can be counted, but with hardly any suggested priorities in terms of technical feasibility, political acceptability, projected cost impact, and health outcomes. Nor has anyone proposed a solid road map to putting the ideas into effect. On the other hand, there are all of the obstacles—cultural, political, professional, and commercial—that stand in the way of implementing those fine ideas (my own included). Our whole health care system is based on a witch's brew of sacrosanct doctor-patient autonomy, a fear of threats to innovation, corporate and (sometimes) physician profit-making, and a belief that, because life is of infinite value, it is morally obnoxious to put a price tag on it.

My political exasperation stems from the fact that neither of the political parties nor any prominent legislator has taken costs on in any serious way. Who wants to lead that kind of crusade? No one, it seems. There has been no shortage of news stories about health care costs and their nasty fallout in personal lives, just as there have also been many foundation reports, at least a few hundred economic studies, and innumerable alarms sounded by federal and state officials about the cost problem. Yet in the decade or so that I have been working on that problem I can discern hardly any significant change in the seemingly inexorable upward slope of costs, any diminishment in the use of old technologies or the introduction of new ones, and—worst of all—no increased sense of urgency about costs, at least if measured by the ultimate test, action.

It was also exasperating during the presidential campaign to hear frequent references to universal care as the Democrat's position and cost control as the Republican stance. There was surely something to that perception if one compared the reform proposals pushed by the candidates from the different parties. But it was hard to escape noticing that, for the Republicans, cost control seemed mainly a stalking horse for expanded privatization of health care. There was no hint that pressure would be brought to bear on the medical drug and device industry or the health care insurers, to rein in their prices and to lower their profit margins. But it was hardly less noticeable that the Democratic candidates went nowhere near confessing that universal care, to be economically affordable and sustainable in the future, would entail rationing and budget limits—and they were all too quick to push improved competition as an important way of controlling costs, a false friend of economic discipline in heath care.

Now I come to the hardest part: moral anguish. It is all too easy for me to sound at least hard-nosed and at worst "cruel and heartless" (as more than a few people have told me) when arguing in favor of drastic financial surgery to cut costs. How can one even think of denying people needed medical care in the name of something so crass as money, and in an affluent society? A question of the kind touches on an old and vexed problem in fashioning public policy: to what extent can public policy, aiming at the common, public good, be reconciled with the individual pain that that the former may entail? The loss of statistical lives, of those people unknown to us and without names, is far easier to accept than the death of those with faces. But once we have seen those faces, of our own family members or friends, and even of strangers, it is a different story. It hurts to imagine denying them what they need. And it can leave me feeling morally shoddy for even moving in that direction, trapped by taking my perception of the gravity of the cost problem seriously.

I was reminded of that feeling just as I was finishing this book. The *New York Times*, in early December 2008, published a long story about a controversial case in the United Kingdom.[1] The British National Health Service had denied an expensive drug, Sutent, to a man Bruce Hardy, dying of disseminated kidney cancer. The cost of that drug was deemed too costly by NICE to be covered—$54,000 for a six-month delay in the progression of the cancer, but not a cure. A public outcry has led the NHS to reconsider its decision. "It's hard to know that there is something out there," his wife said, "that could help but they're saying you can't have it because of cost." I have commended NICE in this book and its use of QALYs (surely brought to bear in this case), but of course if economic standards of that kind are used, and limits are set on treatments, this is exactly the kind of outcry that will follow.

There was one silver lining mentioned in the *Times* story, that of the public pressure it has put on the pharmaceutical companies to lower their prices and work more closely with government to avoid nasty conflicts. There can be little doubt that the United States drug industry will be under considerable pressure in coming years to lower its prices and maybe, just maybe, to tolerate some price controls. The "threat to innovation" argument may be losing its force as a reason to keep prices high—all those future (but not present) lives to be saved.

The trajectory of cancer care stands as a perfect emblem of the profound dilemma of the cost control problem, one that—as the European universal care systems makes clear—is every country's awful challenge and not just ours. Mrs. Hardy's lament that "everyone should be allowed to have as much life as they can" has become a universal aim and expectation, and resistance to taking costs into account its twin brother. We know from current American experience that, if a life-saving or life-extending drug is beyond private or Medicare insurance coverage, desperate families will mortgage all they have to obtain it. But no health care system can provide everything that may save or extend a life. The price of drugs can surely be forced down but it is hard to imagine that every new drug of value can be made as cheap as aspirin. One can take industry's defense of the excessively high costs of so many technologies with a big grain of salt, but they will still remain high.

The data on cancer care in the United States are as good a case study as any to bring the moral dilemma to a full boil. There has been a 13% decline in cancer deaths since 1990, but no decline in the cost of cancer care. It is rising in great part because of the cost of keeping cancer patients alive now who would have died in an earlier era. Progress against cancer does not lower costs, it raises them, a particularly vexing feature of medical progress. The cost of colorectal cancer, for instance, is rising despite a decline in new cases, but it rises because of improved survival and the cost that incurs. So, despite a decreasing incidence, the cost of colorectal cancer will increase by 89% between 2000 and 2020.[2]

That combination will put a particular burden on Medicare because colorectal cancer is principally a disease of old age. "Its future burden on the Medicare program," a National Cancer Institute (NCI) study found, "will be substantial as the number of the elderly grows."[3] In 2004, the national cost of cancer care was about $72 billion. It will grow. Another NCI study noted, of cancer more generally, that "costs are more likely to increase at the individual level as new, more advanced, and more expensive treatments are adopted as standards of care."[4] Not only will government costs increase, but so also will out-of-pocket costs, already prohibitive for thousands of Medicare beneficiaries.

I have four female friends who have breast cancer, all of whom are in their late 70s and early 80s, and with each of whom their cancer is in remission. They have all been in and out of treatment (chemotherapy, radiation) for at least five years, running up great expenses in the process (covered mainly by Medicare). But each of them continues to lead an active life, in no hurry to die. They are my known faces, the ones I think about when I write, and they are real. But I know they are no more real, simply because I can not envision them, than the millions of people whom I can not see but whose lives are being threatened by rising and steadily unaffordable costs. The former are vivid, inescapable, while the latter are hazy, less than distinct, hard to call to mind, but no less real.

I will end by noting an omission, a telling one, in an earlier chapter. In chapter 2, I complained about the action of a Democratic Congress in 2008 in refusing to implement a regulation requiring that physician Medicare fees be reduced. I bemoaned the fact that, when they should be cutting Medicare costs, they were helping to keep them rising. And for good measure they added $20 billion in new expenditures.

I failed to note, however, that the additional appropriation was pri-marily for mental health coverage, to bring it up to the standards long used with physical illness. That was a wonderful, long-overdue benefit. But it was not wonderful to increase a Medicare budget that must stop growing. Both judgments seem to me correct, and there may be times when we just have to live with contradictions. There would have been moral anguish in voting against the mental health benefit and, I would hope, anguish in pushing the Medicare budget in the wrong direction. I do not believe that we can continue to have it both ways, which has been the point of this book, but in this case I am glad it happened. But that has to be the end of it.

NOTES

INTRODUCTION

1. Joseph P. Newhouse, "Medical Care: How Much Welfare Loss?" *Journal of Economic Perspectives* 6, no. 3 (1992): 3–21; Thomas Bodenheimer, "High and Rising Health Care Costs. Part 2: Technologic Innovation," *Annals of Internal Medicine* 142, no. 11 (2005): 932–937; Congressional Budget Office, *Technological Change and the Growth of Health Care Spending* (Washington, D.C.: Congressional Budget Office, 2008); Micah Hartman et al., "U.S. Health Spending by Age, Selected Years Through 2004," *Health Affairs* (Web Exclusive, 2007): W1–W12. A 1998 study summarized the findings of 12 studies between 1971 and 1998 detailing the impact of technology on cost growth: M. E. Chernew et al., "Managed Care, Medical Technology and Health Care Cost Growth: A Review of the Evidence," *Medical Care Research and Review* 55, no. 3 (1998): 274–275; E. A. Peden and M. S. Freeland, "A Historical Analysis of Medical Spending Growth, 1960–1993," *Health Affairs* 14 (1995): 235–247.

2. Sean Keehan et al., "Health Spending Projections Through 2017: The Baby Boom Generation Is Coming to Medicare," *Health Affairs* (Web Exclusive, 2008): W145–155.

3. Quoted in Gardiner Harris, "British Balance Benefit vs. Cost of Latest Drugs," *The New York Times*, December 3, 2008: A1.

4. Ezekiel J. Emanuel and Victor R. Fuchs, "The Perfect Storm of Overutilization," *JAMA* 29, no. 23 (2008): 2789–94.

5. Cathy Schoen et al., "How Many Are Underinsured? Trends among U.S. Adults, 2003 and 2007," *Health Affairs* (Web Exclusive, 2008): W298–W309.

6. Kaiser Family Foundation, "Comparing Projected Growth in Health Care Expenditures and the Economy," In *Snapshots: Health Care Costs* (Menlo Park, CA: Kaiser Family Foundation, 2006).

7. See particularly Paul B. Ginsburg, "Health and Rising Health Care Costs," (Princeton: The Robert Wood Johnson Foundation, Synthesis Report no. 16, November 6, 2008).

CHAPTER 1: MEDICARE ON THE ROPES

1. Congressional Budget Office, *Technological Change and the Growth of Health Care Spending* (Washington, D.C.: Congressional Budget Office, 2008).

2. E.A. Powell, "Fidelity: Couple Needs $225,000 to Cover Health Care in Retirement," *AP Business Wire,* March 5, 2008.

3. Marilyn Moon, "Confronting the Rising Costs of Healthcare and Medicaid," *Generations* (Spring 2005): 62–63.

4. Christine K. Cassell, *Medicare Matters: What Geriatric Medicine Can Teach American Health Care* (Berkeley: University of California Press, 2005): 18.

5. Muriel Gillick, *The Denial of Aging: Perpetual Youth, Eternal Life, and Other Dangerous Fantasies* (Cambridge: Harvard University Press, 2006): 94; Robert A. Berenson and Jane Horvath, "Confronting the Barriers to Chronic Management in Medicare," *Health Affairs* (Web Exclusive, 2002): W3–37–53.

6. David A. Hyman, "Medicare Meets Mephistopheles," *Washington and Lee Law Review* 50, no. 4 (2003): 1184.

7. Jonathan Oberlander, *The Political Life of Medicare* (Chicago: University of Chicago Press, 2003): 4.

8. Ibid., 43–44.

9. Bruce C. Vladeck, "The Struggle for the Soul of Medicare," *Journal of Law, Medicine and Ethics* 32, no. 3 (2004): 412.

10. Hyman, "Medicare Meets Mephistopheles," 1201.

11. Cassell, *Medicare Matters,* 18.

12. "Medicare 'Drifting Toward Disaster': U.S. Official," *Reuters,* April 29, 2008.

13. Peter S. Heller, *Who Will Pay? Coping with Aging Societies, Climate Change, and Other Long-Term Fiscal Responsibilities* (Washington, D.C.: International Monetary Fund, 2003): 222.

14. Federal Hospital Insurance and Federal Supplementary Medical Insurance Trust Funds Board of Trustees, *2008 Annual Report* (Washington, D.C.: Government Printing Office, 2008): 3–4.

15. Ibid., 10.

16. Congressional Budget Office, *The Long-Term Budget Outlook* (Washington, D.C.: Congressional Budget Office: 2003): 29–30.

17. Geoffrey Kollmann and Dawn Nuschler, "The Financial Outlook for Social Security and Medicare," *CRS Report for Congress* (Washington, D.C.: Congressional Research Service, 2004): CRS 1–6.

18. Ibid., 1.

19. Ibid., 6.

20. Oberlander, *The Political Life of Medicare,* 93–95.

21. Marilyn Moon, *Medicare: A Policy Primer* (Washington, D.C.: The Urban Institute Press, 2006): 163.

22. Oberlander, *The Political Life of Medicare,* 99.

23. Congressional Budget Office, *The Long-Term Budget Outlook,* 32.

24. Ibid., 32.

25. Jill Bernstein and Rosemary A. Stevens, "Public Opinion, Knowledge, and Medicare Reform," *Health Affairs* 8, no. 1 (1999): 188–189.

26. Greg M. Shaw and Sarah E. Mysiewicz, "Social Security and Medicare," *Public Opinion Quarterly* 68, no. 3 (2004): 416.

27. Becky Bright, "Reducing Uninsured Seen as Top Health Care Issue, Poll Finds," *Wall Street Journal*, October 24, 2006.

28. Bernstein and Stevens, "Public Opinion, Knowledge, and Medicare Reform," 190–191.

29. Kaiser Family Foundation Public Opinion and Survey Research Program, "Kaiser Health Tracking Poll: Election 2008—April 2008," http://www.kff.org/kaiserpolls/h08-_pomr042908pkg.cfm/.

30. Lewis Thomas, *The Lives of a Cell* (New York: Bantam Books, 1974).

31. BlueCross BlueShield Association, *Medical Cost Reference Guide 2008* (Chicago: BlueCross BlueShield Association, 2008): 49.

32. James F. Fries, "The Compression of Morbidity," *Milbank Quarterly* 61, no. 3 (1983): 347–419.

33. Congressional Budget Office, *Technological Change*, 13.

34. Alan M. Garber and Dana P. Goldman, "The Changing Face of Health Care," in *Coping With Methuselah: The Impact of Molecular Biology on Medicine and Society*, ed. Henry J. Aaron and William B. Schwartz (Washington, D.C.: Brookings Institution Press, 2004): 111; Dana P. Goldman et al., "Consequences of Health Trends and Medical Innovation for the Future Elderly," *Health Affairs* 24, suppl. 2 (2005): R5–17.

35. David M. Cutler, Allison B. Rosen, and Sandeep Vijan, "The Value of Medical Spending in the United States, 1960–2000," *New England Journal of Medicine* 355, no. 9 (2006): 923.

36. Ibid.

37. Jonathan Skinner and Elliott S. Fisher, *The Efficiency of Medicare* (Cambridge, MA: National Bureau of Economics, 2001): 22.

38. Goldman, "Consequences of Health Trends and Medical Innovation for the Future Elderly," R5–R16.

39. Geoffrey F. Joyce et al., "The Lifetime Burden of Chronic Disease among the Elderly," *Health Affairs* 24, supplement 2 (2005): R18–R29; Michael Chernew et al., "Barriers to Constructing Health Care Cost Growth," *Health Affairs* 23, no. 6 (2004): 122–128; Jayanta Bhattacharya et al., "Technological Advances in Cancer and Future Spending by the Elderly," *Health Affairs* 24, supplement 2 (2005): R53–R56; James Lubitz, "Health, Technology, and Medical Spending," *Health Affairs* 24, web exclusive 2 (2005): 83.

40. Darios K. Lakdawalla, Dana P. Goldman, and Baoping Shang, "The Health and Cost Consequences of Obesity among the Future Elderly," *Health Affairs* 24, supplement 2 (2005): R30.

41. Bhattacharya et al., "Technological Advances," R53–R56.

42. David M. Cutler, "The Potential for Cost Savings in Medicare's Future," *Health Affairs* 24, supplement 2 (2005): WR-R78.

43. Cassell, *Medicare Matters*, 198, 41.

44. Joseph White, *False Alarm: Why the Greatest Threat to Social Security and Medicare Is the Campaign to "Save" Them* (Baltimore: The Johns Hopkins University Press, 2001): 2.

45. Ibid., 8.

46. Laura McGinley, "A Guide to Who Wins and Who Loses in Medicare Bill," *Wall Street Journal*, November 18, 2003.

47. Dick Armey, "Say 'No' to the Medicare Bill," *Wall Street Journal*, November 21, 2003.

48. Regina Herzlinger, *Who Killed Health Care? America's $2 Trillion Medical Problem—and the Consumer-Driven Cure* (New York: McGraw-Hill, 2007).

49. Kenneth G. Manton, XiLiang Gu, and Vicki L. Lamb, "Long-Term Trends in Life Expectancy and Active Life Expectancy in the United States," *Population and Development Review* 32, no. 1 (2006): 81–105; Alicia H. Munnell, Robert E. Hatch, and James G. Lee, *Why Is Life Expectancy So Low in the United States?* (Boston: Center for Retirement Research, 2001), http://crr.bc.edu/briefs/why_is_life_expectancy_so_low_in_the_united_states_.html/.

50. The Heritage Foundation, "Lessons of Success: What Congress Can Learn from the Federal Employees Program," Robert E. Moffit, http://www.heritage.org/Research/HealthCare/wm565.cfm; Walton Francis, *Using the Federal Employees' Model: Nine Tests for Rational Medicare Reform: Heritage Foundation Backgrounder #1675* (Washington, D.C.: The Heritage Foundation, 2003); David Gratzer, *The Cure: How Capitalism Can Save American Health Care* (New York: Encounter Books, 2006): 133–137.

51. Greg Scandlen, "Defined Contribution Health Insurance," *Policy Backgrounder*, no. 15 (Washington, D.C.: Center for Policy Analysis, 2000).

52. Ezekial J. Emanuel and Victor R. Fuchs, "Health Care Vouchers—A Proposal for Universal Coverage," *New England Journal of Medicine* 352, no. 12 (2005): 1255.

53. Brian Biles, Emily Adrion, Stuart Guterman, "The Continuing Costs of Privatization: Extra Payments to Medicare Advantage," e-alert, The Commonwealth Fund, September 5, 2008.

54. Marilyn Moon, *Medicare: A Policy Primer*, 100.

55. Mark Schlesinger, "Markets as Belief Systems and Those Who Keep the Faith," *Journal of Health Politics, Policy, and Law* 31, no. 3 (2006): 417–421; Theodore R. Marmor, *The Politics of Medicare, 2nd edition* (New York: Aldine Transaction, 2000).

56. Sarah Thomson and Elias Mossialos, *What are the Equity, Efficiency and Choice Implications of Private Health-Care Funding in Western Europe?* (Copenhagen: World Health Organization Regional Office for Europe, 2004):10.

57. Ibid., 12.

58. Ibid.

59. Ibid.

60. Ibid.

61. Kaiser Family Foundation, "Comparing Projected Growth in Health Care Expenditures and the Economy," in *Snapshots: Health Care Costs* (Menlo Park, CA: Kaiser Family Foundation, 2006): 3.

62. Ibid., 5.

63. Sherry Glied, "Health Care Costs on the Rise Again," *Journal of Economic Perspectives* 17, no. 2 (2003): 145.

64. Moon, *Medicare Matters*, 164.

65. Vladeck, "The Struggle for the Soul of Medicare," 415.

CHAPTER 2: TAMING THE BELOVED BEAST:
MEDICAL TECHNOLOGY

1. Daniel Callahan, "How Much Is Enough or Too Little: Assessing Health Care Demand in Developed Countries," in *Comprehensive Medicinal Chemistry II*, vol. 1, ed. John B. Taylor and David J. Triggle (Amsterdam: Elsevier, 2007): 627–636.

2. Ibid.

3. Kaiser Family Foundation, "Health Care Spending in the United States and OECD Countries," in *Snapshots: Health Care Costs* (Menlo Park, CA: Kaiser Family Foundation, 2007), http://www.kff.org/insurance/snapshot/chcm010307oth.cfm/.

4. Kenneth E. Thorpe, *Impact on Health Care Reform: Projections of Cost and Savings* (Washington, D.C.: National Coalition on Health Care, 2005).

5. Alan B. Cohen and Ruth S. Hanft, ed., *Technology in American Health Care* (Ann Arbor: University of Michigan, 2004): 19; Joseph P. Newhouse, "Medicare Spending on Physicians—No Easy Fix in Sight," *New England Journal of Medicine* 356, no. 18 (2007): 1883–1884.

6. Patrice Bourdelais, *Epidemics Laid Low: A History of What Happened in Rich Countries*, trans. Bart K. Holland (Baltimore: Johns Hopkins University Press, 2006): 138.

7. Ibid., 139.

8. Richard White, "The Nature of Progress: Progress and the Environment," in *Progress: Fact or Illusion?*, ed. Leo Marx and Bruce Mazlish (Ann Arbor, University of Michigan Press, 1996): 134.

9. Richard D. Lamm and Robert H. Blank, *Condition Critical: A New Moral Vision for Health Care* (Golden, CO: Fulcrum Publishing, 2007).

10. Alastair J. J. Wood, "When Increased Therapeutic Benefit Comes at Increased Cost," *New England Journal of Medicine* 346, no. 23 (2002): 1820.

11. Marjorie E. Ginsburg, "A Survey of Physician Attitudes and Practices Concerning Cost-Effectiveness in Patient Care," *Western Journal of Medicine* 173, no. 6 (2000): 392.

12. Ibid.

13. Henry J. Aaron and William B. Schwartz, *Can We Say No? The Challenge of Rationing Health Care* (Washington, D.C.: The Brookings Institution Press, 2005): 6.

14. Ibid., 7.

15. Alan M. Garber and Dana P. Goldman, "The Changing Face of Health Care," in *Coping With Methuselah: The Impact of Molecular Biology on Medicine and Society*, ed. Henry J. Aaron and William B. Schwartz (Washington, D.C.: Brookings Institution Press, 2004): 123.

16. Robert J. Samuelson, "The Medicare Monster," *The Washington Post*, September 14, 2006; Henry J. Aaron, "The Unsurprising Surprise of Renewed Health Care Cost Inflation," *Health Affairs* (Web Exclusive, 2002): W85–W87.

17. Tyler Cowen, "Poor U.S. Scores in Health Care Don't Measure Nobels and Innovation," *New York Times*, December 3, 2007.

18. Molly J. Coye and Jason Kell, "How Hospitals Confront New Technology," *Health Affairs* 25, no. 1 (2006): 163; Barry M. Straube, "How Changes in the Medicare Coverage Process Have Facilitated the Spread of New Technologies," *Health Affairs* (Web Exclusive, 2005): W314–W316.

19. Susan B. Foote, *Managing the Medicare Arms Race: Public Policy and Medical Device Innovation* (Berkeley: University of California Press, 1992).

20. Jacqueline Fox, "Medicare Should, but Cannot, Consider Cost: Legal Impediments to a Sound Policy," *Buffalo Law Review* 53, no. 2 (2005): 577–633; Susan B. Foote and Lynn A. Blewett, "Politics of Prevention: Expanding Prevention Benefits in the Medicare Program," *Journal of Public Health Policy* 24, no. 1 (2003): 26–40; Sean R. Tunis, "Why Medicare Has Not Established Criteria for Coverage Decisions," *New England Journal of Medicine* 350, no. 21 (2004): 2196–2198; Peter J. Neumann, *Using Cost-Effective Analysis to Improve Health Care* (New York: Oxford University Press, 2005).

21. Muriel R. Gillick, "Molecular Medicine, The Medicare Drug Benefit, and the Need for Cost Control," *Journal of the American Geriatrics Society* 54, no. 9 (2006): 1442–1446.

22. Henry J. Aaron, "Should Public Policy Seek to Control the Growth of Health Care Spending?" *Health Affairs* (Web Exclusive, 2003): W3–W31.

23. Minah Kim, Robert J. Blendon, and John M. Benson, "How Interested Are Americans in New Medical Technologies?" *Health Affairs* 20, no. 5 (2001): 194–201.

24. Ibid.

25. Ibid., 200.

26. Ibid., 201.

27. Janet K. Shim, Ann J. Russ, and Sharon R. Kaufman, "Risk, Life Extension and the Pursuit of Medical Possibility," *Sociology of Health and Illness* 38, no. 4 (2006): 479–502.

28. Ibid., 483.

29. Ibid., 490.

30. Carol J. DeFrances and Margaret J. Hall, "2005 National Hospital Discharge Survey," *Advance Data from Vital and Health Statistics* 385 (Centers for Disease Control and Prevention, 2007): 1; Sharon R. Kaufman, *And a Time to Die: How American Hospitals Shape the End of Life* (Chicago: University of Chicago Press, 2005).

31. Michael Chernew et al. "Barriers to Constraining Health Care Cost Growth," *Health Affairs* 23, no. 6 (2004): 123.

32. Ibid., 125.

33. Ibid., 126.

34. Susan B. Foote and Robert J. Town, "Implementing Evidence-Based Medicine through Medicine Coverage Decisions," *Health Affairs* 26, no. 6 (2007): 1634–1642.

35. Daniel Callahan, *What Price Better Health? Hazards of the Research Imperative* (Berkeley: University of California Press, 2006): 223–233.

36. Congressional Budget Office, *Technological Change and the Growth of Health Care Spending* (Washington, D.C.: Congressional Budget Office, 2008): 13.

37. H. Gilbert Welch et al., "What's Making Us Sick Is an Epidemic of Diagnoses," *New York Times*, January 2, 2007.

38. Laura A. Dummit, "Medicare Physician Payments and Spending," in *National Health Policy Forum*, Issue brief 185 (Washington, D.C.: The George Washington University Press, 2006): 4; Barbara M. Rothenberg, *Medical Technology as a Driver of Health Care Costs: Diagnostic Imaging* (Washington, D.C.: BlueCross BlueShield Association, 2003), http://www.bcbs.com/betterknowledge/cost/diagnostic-imaging.html; H. Gilbert Welch, *Should I Be Tested for Cancer?* (Berkeley: University of California Press, 2004).

39. Dummit, "Medicare Physician Payments and Spending," 4.

40. Julie Appleby, "The Case of CT Angiography: How Americans View and Embrace New Technology," *Health Affairs* 27, no. 6 (2008): 1515–21.

41. Coye and Kell, "How Hospitals Confront New Technology," 165.

42. Ibid., 166.

43. Ibid., 172.

44. Jeff Goldsmith, "Technology and the Boundaries of the Hospital: Three Emerging Technologies," *Health Affairs* 23, no. 6 (2004): 150.

45. Laurence Baker et al., "The Relationship between Technology Availability and Health Care Spending," *Health Affairs* (Web Exclusive, 2003): W537–W551.

46. Patricia M. Danzon and Mark V. Pauly, "Insurance and New Technology: From Hospital to Drugstore," *Health Affairs* 20, no. 5 (2005): 86–100.

47. Cindy L. Bryce and Ellen Cline, "The Supply and Use of Selected Medical Technologies," *Health Affairs* 17, no. 1 (1998): 221.

48. Muriel R. Gillick, "The Technological Imperative and the Battle for the Hearts of America," *Perspectives in Biology and Medicine* 50, no. 2 (2007): 276–294.

49. Aaron and Schwartz, *Can We Say No?*, 90.

50. Alan B. Cohen and Ruth S. Hanft, "Evaluation Concerns: Medical Technology Evaluation in the Future," in *Technology in American Health Care* ed. Alan B. Cohen and Ruth S. Hanft (Ann Arbor: University of Michigan, 2004): 364.

51. Joseph P. Newhouse, *Free for All? Lessons from The Rand Health Insurance Experiment* (Cambridge: Harvard University Press, 1993).

52. Joshua T. Cohen, Peter J. Neumann, and Milton C. Weinstein, "Does Prevention Save Money? Health Economics and the Presidential Candidates," *New England Journal of Medicine* 358, no. 7 (2008): 661–663.

53. Klim McPherson, "Does Preventing Obesity Lead to Reduced Health-Care Costs?" *PLoS Medicine* 5, no. 2 (2008): e37.

54. David M. Eddy, "Evidence-Based Medicine: A Unified Approach," *Health Affairs* 24, no. 1 (2005): 9.

55. Jill Eden et al., *Knowing What Works in Health Care: A Roadmap for the Nation* (Washington, D.C.: National Academies Press, 2008).

56. Uwe Reinhardt, "An Information Infrastructure for the Pharmaceutical Market," *Health Affairs* 23, no. 1 (2004): 107–112.

57. Stefan Timmermans and Aaron Mauck, "The Promise and Pitfalls of Evidence-Based Medicine," *Health Affairs* 24, no. 1 (2005): 18–28; Dan Mendelson and Tanisha V. Carino, "Evidence-Based Medicine in the United States—De Rigueur or Dream Deferred?" *Health Affairs* 24, no. 1 (2005): 133–136; Eddy, "Evidence-Based Medicine," 9–17; Andrew Miles, Andreas Polychronis, and Joseph E. Grey, "The Evidence-Based Health Care Debate," *Journal of Evaluation in Clinical Practice* 12, no. 3 (2006): 239–247.

58. Gerard F. Anderson et al., "Health Care Spending and Use of Information Technology in OECD Countries," *Health Affairs* 25, no. 3 (2006): 819–831.

59. Rand Corporation, "Health Information Technology: Can HIT Lower Costs and Improve Technology?" in *Rand Health: Research Highlights* (Santa Monica: Rand Corporation, 2005).

60. Rainu Kaushal et al., "The Costs of a National Health Information Network," *Annals of Internal Medicine* 143, no. 3 (2005): 165–173.

61. Anderson et al., "Health Care Spending," 828.

62. Steven Lohr, "Smart Care Via a Mouse, but What Will It Cost?" *New York Times*, August 20, 2006.

63. National Conference of State Legislatures, "Certificate of Need: State Health Laws and Programs," (November 17, 2008); http://www.ncsl.org/programs/health/cert-need.htm.

64. Andrew Chernew, Richard A. Hirth, and Seema S. Sonnad, "Managed Care, Medical Technology, and Health Care Cost Growth," *Medical Care Research and Review* 55, no. 3 (1998): 259–288.

65. Karen Davis et al., *Slowing the Growth of U.S. Health Care Expenditures: What Are the Options?* (New York: The Commonwealth Fund, 2007).

66. Cathy Schoen et al., "Bending the Curve: Options for a Achieving Savings and Improving Value in U.S. Health Spending," *The Commonwealth Fund* 80 (2007).

67. Joseph R. Antos and Alice M. Rivlin, ed., "Strategies for Slowing the Growth of Health Spending," in *Restoring Fiscal Sanity 2007: The Health Spending Challenge* (Washington, D.C.: The Brookings Institution Press, 2007): 28–80.

68. Kenneth E. Thorpe and David H. Howard, "The Rise in Spending among Medicare Beneficiaries: The Role of Chronic Disease Prevalence and Changes in Treatment Intensity," *Health Affairs* (Web Exclusive, 2006): W378–W388.

69. Ibid., W385.

70. Ibid., W386.

71. Dana P. Goldman and Neeraj Sood, "Rising Medicare Costs: Are We in Crisis?" *Health Affairs* (Web Exclusive, 2006): W390.

72. Ibid., W392.

CHAPTER 3: GETTING SERIOUS ABOUT COSTS AND TECHNOLOGY

1. Obama '08, "Barack Obama's Plan for a Healthy America: Lowering Health Care Costs and Ensuring Affordable, High-Quality Health Care for All," http://www.barackobama.com/pdf/issues/HealthCareFullPlan.pdf.

2. Max Baucus, "Health Care Reform 2009," (Washington, D.C.: Senate Finance Committee, November 12, 2008).

3. Thomas Daschle, Critical: What Can We Do About the Health Care Crisis (New York: St. Martin's Press, 2008).

4. The Healthy Americans Act, HR 3163, 110th Congress.

5. Ibid.

6. National Coalition on Health Care, Building a Better Health Care System: Specifications for Reform (Washington, D.C.: National Coalition on Health Care, 2004).

7. Donald J. Palmisano, David W. Emmons, and Gregory D. Wozniak, "Expanding Insurance Coverage through Tax Credits, Consumer Choice, and Market Enhancements: The American Medical Association Proposal for Health Insurance Reform," JAMA 291, no. 18 (2004): 2237–42.

8. Victor R. Fuchs and Ezekiel J. Emanuel, "Health Care Reform: Why? What? When?" Health Affairs 24, no. 6 (2005): 1399–1414; Ezekiel J. Emanuel, Health Care Guaranteed (New York: Public Affairs, 2008).

9. Kaiser Family Foundation, "Kaiser Health Tracking Poll: Election 2008," http://www.kff.org/kaiserpolls/upload/7807.pdf/.

10. Editorial, "The Battle Over Health Care," New York Times, September 23, 2007; Dallas L. Salisbury, "Tough Choices Ahead: Candidates Ignore Pain of Needed Cuts to Health Care," The Commonwealth Fund (January 2008).

11. Richard B. Saltman, "Melting Public-Private Boundaries in European Health Systems," The European Journal of Public Health 13, no. 1 (2003): 24–29.

12. Richard B. Saltman and Josep Figueras, European Health Care Reform: Analysis of Current Strategies (Copenhagen: WHO Regional Publications, 1997): 100.

13. Ibid.; AARP, European Experiences with Health Care Cost Containment: France, The Netherlands, Norway, and The United Kingdom (Washington, D.C.: AARP, 2006), http://assets.aarp.org/www.aarp.org_/cs/gap/ldrstudy_costcontain.pdf.

14. Saltman and Figueras, European Health Care Reform; Richard B. Saltman, Reinhard Busse, and Josep Figueras, Social Insurance Systems in Western Europe (Maidenhead, U.K.: Open University Press, 2004).

15. Corina Sorenson, Michael Drummond, and Panos Kavanos, "Ensuring Value for Money in Health Care: The Role of Health Technology Assessment in the European Union," European Observatory Series, no. 11 (Copenhagen: WHO Regional Office for Europe, 2008).

16. Elias Mossialos, Monique Mrazek, and Tom Walley, ed., Regulating Pharmaceuticals in Europe: Striving for Efficiency, Equity, and Quality (Maidenhead, U.K., Open University Press, 2004); Organization for Economic Cooperation and Development, Health at a Glance: OECD Indicators 2003 (Paris: OECD, 2003).

17. Technological Change in Health Care Research Network, "Technological Change Around the World: Evidence from Heart Attack Care," *Health Affairs* 20, no. 30 (2001): 25–42.

18. Organization for Economic Cooperation and Development, *Projecting OECD Health and Long-Term Care Expenditures: What Are the Main Drivers?* (Paris: OECD, 2006), *http://www.oecd.org/dataoecd/57/7/36085940.pdf/*.

19. Gerard F. Anderson et al., "It's the Prices Stupid: Why the United States Is So Different from Other Countries," *Health Affairs* 22, no. 3 (2003): 101.

20. Robert G. Evans et al., "The 20 Year Experiment: Accounting for, Explaining, and Evaluating Health Care Cost Containment in Canada and the United States," *Annual Review of Public Health* 12 (1991): 481–518.

21. *The National Health Insurance Act*, HR 676, 110th Congress.

22. The Physicians Working Group for Single-Payer National Health Insurance, "Proposal of the Physicians' Working Group for Single-Payer National Health Insurance," *JAMA* 290, no. 6 (2003): 798–805.

23. Ibid., 801.

24. Robert J. Blendon and Karen Donelan, "The Public and the Emerging Debate over National Health Insurance," *New England Journal of Medicine* 323, no. 3 (1990).

25. Robert J. Blendon and John M. Benson, "Americans' Views on Health Policy: A Fifty-Year Historical Perspective," *Health Affairs* 20, no. 2 (2001): 33–46.

26. Robert J. Blendon et al., "The Implications of the 1992 Presidential Election for Health Care Reform," *JAMA* 268, no. 23 (1993): 3373.

27. Jennifer P. Ruger, "Health, Health Care, and Incompletely Theorized Agreements: A Normative Theory of Health Policy Decision Making," *Journal of Health Politics, Policy and Law* 32, no. 1 (2007): 74.

28. Jill Quadagno, *One Nation Uninsured: Why the U.S. Has No National Health Insurance* (New York: Oxford University Press, 2005).

29. David M. Cutler, *Your Money or Your Life: Strong Medicine for America's Health Care System* (New York: Oxford University Press, 2004): 62.

30. Daniel Callahan, "Using Humans for Research," in *What Price Better Health: Hazards of the Research Imperative* (Berkeley: University of California Press, 2003).

31. Jack E. Triplett, ed., *Measuring the Prices of Medical Treatments* (Washington, D.C.: The Brookings Institution Press, 1999); Kevin A. Murphy and Robert H. Topel, *Measuring the Gains from Medical Research: An Economic Approach* (Chicago: The University of Chicago Press, 2003).

32. Josep Figueras et al., *Health Systems, Health, and Wealth: Assessing the Case for Investing in Health* (Copenhagen: World Health Organization and the European Observatory, 2008): 65.

33. Ibid., 5.

34. Stephen Martin, Nigel Rice, and Peter C. Smith, "Does Health Care Spending Improve Health Outcomes? Evidence from English Programme Budgeting Data," *Journal of Health Economics* 27, no. 4 (2008): 826–42.

35. Gina Kolata, "Co-Payments Go Way Up for Drugs with High Prices," *New York Times*, April 14, 2008.

36. United Health Foundation, *America's Health Rankings 2005* (Washington, D.C.: United Health Foundation, 2005), *http://www.unitedhealthfoundation.org/shr2005/ahr05_email.pdf*.

37. Alan Garber, Dana P. Goldman, and Anupam B. Jena, "The Promise of Health Care Cost Containment," *Health Affairs* 26, no. 6 (2007): 1545–47.

38. Henry J. Aaron and William B. Schwartz, *Can We Say No? The Challenge of Rationing Health Care* (Washington, D.C.: The Brookings Institution Press, 2005): 3.

39. Corina Sorenson, Michael Drummond, and Panos Kavanos, "Ensuring Value for Money in Health Care: The Role of Health Technology Assessment in the European Union," *European Observatory Series* no. 11 (Copenhagen: WHO Regional Office for Europe, 2008). See also Marcial Velasco Garrido, et al. "Health Technology Assesment and Health Policy-Making in Europe," *European Observatory Series No. 14* (Copenhagen: WHO Regional Office for Europe, 2008).

40. Ibid., 5.

41. Ibid., 9.

42. David Meltzer, "Can Medical Cost-Effectiveness Analysis Identify the Value of Research?" in *Measuring the Gains from Medical Research: An Economic Approach*, ed. Kevin A. Murphy and Robert H. Topel (Chicago: The University of Chicago Press): 211.

43. Corina Sorenson et al, "Ensuring Value for Money in Health Care"; see also, Drew Laughland et al., "Exploring the Role of Cost–benefit Analysis in Government Regulations," *AARP Public Policy Institute* (Washington, D.C.: AARP, 2007).

44. Marthe Gold, "Panel on Cost-Effectiveness in Health and Medicine," *Medical Care* 34, no. 12 (1996) supplement: DS197-DS199.

45. John Harris, "NICE Is Not Cost Effective," *Journal of Medical Ethics* 32, no. 7 (2006): 378–380; Karl Claxton and Anthony J. Culyer, "Rights, Responsibilities, and NICE: A Rejoinder to Harris," *Journal of Medical Ethics* 33, no. 8 (2007): 462–64; Peter H. Schuck and Richard J. Zeckhauser, *Targeting in Social Programs* (Washington, D.C.: The Brookings Institution Press, 2006).

46. Norman Daniels and James E. Sabin, *Setting Limits Fairly: Can We Learn to Share Medical Resources?* (New York: Oxford University Press, 2000); Madison Powers and Ruth Faden, "Setting Priorities," in *Social Justice: The Moral Foundations of Public Health and Health Policy* (New York: Oxford University Press, 2006).

47. Alan Maynard, "Rationing Health Care: An Exploration," *Health Policy* 49, no. 1–2 (1999): 5–11.

48. Elias Mossialos and Derek King, "Citizens and Rationing: Analysis of a European Survey," *Health Policy* 49, no. 1–2 (1999): 75–135.

49. Ibid., 98.

50. Ibid., 113.

CHAPTER 4: COMPETITION: THE FIX THAT WILL FAIL

1. Kenneth J. Arrow, "Uncertainty and the Welfare Economics of Medical Care," *The American Economics Review* 53, no. 5 (1963): 941–973.
2. Burton Weisbrod, "Competition in Health Care: A Cautionary View," in *Market Reforms in Health Care: Current Issues, New Directions*, ed. Jack Meyers (Washington, D.C.: AEI Press, 1983): 71.
3. James C. Robinson, "The End of Asymmetric Information," *Journal of Health Politics, Policy, and Law* 26, no. 5 (2001): 1045.
4. Thomas Rice, "Can Markets Give Us the Health System We Want?" *Journal of Health Politics, Policy, and Law* 22, no. 2 (1997): 384.
5. Thomas Rice, *The Economics of Health Reconsidered*, 2nd ed. (Chicago: Health Administration Press, 2002): 6.
6. Ibid., 422–423.
7. Mark V. Pauly, "Who Was That Straw Man Anyway? A Comment on Evans and Rice," *Journal of Health Politics, Policy, and Law* 22, no. 2 (1997): 470.
8. Stuart Butler and Edmund Haislmaier, *A National Health System for America* (Washington, D.C.: The Heritage Foundation Press, 1989).
9. Alain Enthoven, "Introducing Market Forces in Health Care: A Tale of Two Countries" (paper presented at the Fourth European Conference on Health Economics, Paris, France, July 10, 2002).
10. Stephen M. Davidson et al., "Competition and Quality among Managed Care Plans in the U.S.A.," *International Journal for Quality in Health Care* 10, no. 5 (1998): 411–419.
11. Jonathan Gruber, "The Effect of Competitive Pressure on Charity: Hospital Responses to Price Shopping in California." *Journal of Health Economics* 13, no. 2 (1994): 183–212.
12. Patrick A. Rivers, Saundra Glover, George Monchus, "Hospital Competition in Major U.S. Metropolitan Areas: Empirical Evidence," *Journal of Health and Health Services Administration*, Summer 2000: 37–49.
13. Harold Luft et al., "Hospital Competition, Cost and Medical Practice," *The Journal of Medical Practice Management* 4, no. 1 (1988): 10–15.
14. Glenn A. Melnick and Jack Zwanziger, "Hospital Behavior under Competition and Cost-Containment Policies: The California Experience, 1980 to 1985," *JAMA* 260, no. 18 (1988): 2669–2675.
15. Thomas L. Gift, Richard Arnould, Larry DeBrock, "Healthy Competition Healthy?" *Inquiry* 39 (2002): 45–55.
16. R. Town and G. Vistnes, "Hospital Competition in HMO Networks." *Journal of Health Economics* 20 (2001): 733–753.
17. Gautam Gowrisankaranand and Robert J. Town, "Competition, Payers, and Hospital Quality," *Health Services Research* 38, no. 6 (2003): 1403–1421.
18. P. A. Rivers and M. D. Fottler, "Do HMO Penetration and Hospital Competition Impact Quality of Hospital Care?" *Health Services Management Research* 17, no. 4 (2004): 237–248.

19. Jeanette Rogowski, Arrind K. Jain, and José J. Escarce, "Hospital Competition, Managed Care, and Mortality after Hospitalization for Medical Conditions in California," *Health Services Research* 42, no. 2 (2007): 682–705.

20. Anil Bemazai, "Price competition and Hospital Cost Growth in the United States (1989–1994)," *Health Economics* 8, no. 3 (1999): 233–243.

21. Emmett B. Keeler, Glenn Melnick, and Jack Zwanziger, "The Changing Effects of Competition on Non-Profit and For-Profit Hospital Pricing Behavior," *Journal of Health Economics* 18, no. 1 (1999): 69–86.

22. Ibid., 83.

23. Thomas Bodenheimer, "High and Rising Health Care Costs. Part I: Seeking an Explanation," *Annals of Internal Medicine* 142, no. 10 (2005): 852.

24. Ibid.

25. James C. Robinson, "Consolidation and the Transformation of Competition in Health Care," *Health Affairs* 23, no. 6 (2004): 20.

26. Bemazai et al., "Price Competition," 233-243.

27. Gerard Anderson, Robert Heyssel, and Robert Dickler, "Competition vs. Regulation: Its Effect on Hospitals." *Health Affairs* 12, no. 1 (1993): 70–80.

28. James C. Robinson and Harold Luft, "Competition, Regulation, and Hospital Costs, 1982 to 1986," *JAMA* 260, no. 18 (1988): 2676–2681.

29. Jack Zwanziger and Glenn A. Melnick, "The Effects of Competition on the Hospital Industry: The Evidence from California," in *Competitive Approaches to Health Care Reform*, ed. Robert J. Arnould, Robert F. Rich, and William D. White (Washington, D.C.: The Urban Institute Press, 1993): 133.

30. Stephen N. Shortell and Edward F. Hughes, "The Effects of Regulation, Competition, and Ownership on Mortality Rates among Hospital Patients," *New England Journal of Medicine* 318, no. 17 (1988): 1100–1107.

31. Rogowski et al., "Hospital Competition," 682–705.

32. Kevin G. Volpe and Edward Buckley, "The Effect of Increases in HMO Penetration and Changes in Payer Mix on In-Hospital Mortality and treatment Patterns for Acute Myocardial Infarction," *The American Journal of Managed Care* 10, no. 7 (2004): 505–512.

33. Douglas A. Wholey, Roger Feldman, and Jon B. Christianson, "The Effect of Market Structure on HMO Premiums," *Journal of Health Economics* 14, no. 1 (1995): 81–105.

34. Barbara A. Mark, David W. Harless, and Michael McCue, "The Impact of HMO Penetration on the Relationship between Nurse Staffing and Quality," *Health Economics* 14, no. 7 (2005): 737–753.

35. Dennis P. Scanlon et al., "Competition and Health Plan Performance: Evidence from Health Maintenance Organization Insurance Markets," *Medical Care* 43, no. 4 (2005): 338–346.

36. Farasat Bokhari, "Managed Care Competition and the Adoption of Hospital Technology: The Case of Cardiac Catheterization," *http://129.3.20.41/eps/hew/papers/0110/0110001.pdf*.

37. Patrick A. Rivers and Myron D. Fottler, "Do HMO Penetration and Hospital Competition Impact Quality of Hospital Care?" *Health Services Management Research* 17, no. 4 (2004): 237–248.

38. Walton Francis, *Using the Federal Employees' Model: Nine Tests for Rational Medicare Reform: Heritage Foundation Backgrounder #1675* (Washington, D.C.: The Heritage Foundation, 2003); David Gratzer, *The Cure: How Capitalism Can Save American Health Care* (New York: Encounter Books, 2006).

39. American Federation of Government Employees, *2007 Issue Paper Federal Employees Health Benefits Program* (Washington, D.C.: AFGE, 2007), *http://www.afge.org/index.cfm?page=ContentTest&Fuse=Content&ContentID=996*.

40. U.S. Office of Personnel Management, "Federal Employees Health Benefits Program," *http://www.opm.gov/insure/health/*.

41. John E. Dicken, Director of Health Care, Government Accountability Office, testimony before the Subcommittee on Oversight of Government Management, Friday, May 18, 2007.

42. John K. Iglehart, "The Emergence of Physician-Owned Specialty Hospitals," *New England Journal of Medicine* 352, no. 1 (2005): 78–84.

43. Medicare Payment Advisory Commission (MEDPAC), *Report to the Congress: Physician-Owned Specialty Hospitals Revisited* (Washington, D.C.: Medicare Payment Advisory Commission, 2006).

44. Robert L. Ohsfeldt and John E. Schneider, *The Business of Health: The Role of Competition, Markets, and Regulation* (Washington, D.C.: AEI Press, 2006).

45. Gratzer, *The Cure*.

46. Frederick T. Schut and Wynand Van de Ven, "Rationing and Competition in the Dutch Health Care System," *Health Economics* 14, supplement 1 (2005): S59. Timothy Stoltzfus Jost, Diane Dawson, Andre de Exter, "The Role of Competition in Health Care: A Western European Perspective," *Journal of Health Politics, Policy and Law* 31, no. 3 (2006): 688–703; Richard Freeman, "Competition in Context: The Politics of Heath Care Reform in Europe," *International Journal for Quality in Health Care* 10, no. 5 (1998): 395–401.

47. Thomas Schlesinger, ed., "Federal Trade Commission Report on Health Care and Competition," special issue, *Journal of Health Politics, Policy, and Law* 31, no. 3 (2006).

48. Alain Enthoven, "A Living Model of Managed Competition: A Conversation with Dutch Health Minister Ab Klink," *Health Affairs*, Web Exclusive (2008): W196–203.

49. Hans Maarse, personal communication, 2007.

50. Paul Vaillancourt Rosenau and Christiaan Lako, "An Experiment with Regulated Competition and Individual Mandates for Universal Health Care: The New Dutch Health Insurance System," *Journal of Health Politics, Policy and Law* 33, no. 6 (2008): 1031.

51. Hans Maarse and Rud Ter Meulen, "Consumer Choice in Dutch Health Insurance after Reform," *Health Care Analysis* 14, no. 1 (2006): 37–49.

52. Timothy S. Jost, "The Future of Medicare, Post Great Society and Post Plus-Choice: Legal and Policy Issues," *Washington and Lee Law Review* 60, no. 4 (2003): 1087–1094.

53. Joseph White, "Markets and Medical Care: The United States, 1993–2005," *The Milbank Quarterly* 85, no. 3 (2007): 432.

54. Michael E. Porter and Elizabeth O. Teisberg, *Redefining Health Care: Creating Value-Based Competition on Results* (Boston: Harvard Business School Press, 2006); Gratzer, *The Cure*; John F. Cogan, R. Glenn Hubbard, Daniel P. Kessler, *Healthy, Wealthy, and Wise: Five Steps to a Better Health Care System* (Washington, D.C.: AEI Press, 2005); Robert L. Ohsfeldt and John E. Schneider, *The Business of Health: The Role of Competition, Markets, and Regulation* (Washington, D.C.: The AEI Press, 2006).

55. Ohsfeldt and Schneider, *The Business of Health.*

56. Michael F. Cannon and Michael D. Tanner, *Healthy Competition: What's Holding Back Health Care and How to Free It* (Washington, D.C.: The Cato Institute, 2005): 5.

57. Ibid., 116.

58. John F. Coogan, R. Glen Hubbard, and Daniel P. Kessler, *Healthy, Wealthy, & Wise* (Washington, D.C.: The AEI Press, 2005).

59. Ibid., 81–82.

60. Porter and Teisberg, *Redefining Health Care.*

61. Hans Maarse, personal communication, 2007.

62. Daniel Callahan and Angela Wassuna, "The Value of the Market: What Does the Evidence Show?" in *Medicine and the Market: Equity v. Choice* (Baltimore: Johns Hopkins University Press, 2006).

63. Jacob S. Hacker, "The Case for Public Health Choice in National Health Reform: Key to Cost Control and Quality Coverage" (Berkeley: Center on Health, Economic & Family Security, University of California, Berkeley, School of Law, December 2008).

CHAPTER 5: THE COHABITATION OF MEDICINE AND COMMERCE

1. Seymour Perry, "The Brief Life of The National Center for Health Care Technology," *New England Journal of Medicine* 307, no. 17 (1982): 1096.

2. Ibid., 1096.

3. Ibid.

4. Ibid., 1098.

5. Ibid.

6. Shannon Brownlee, *Overtreated: Why Too Much Medicine Is Making Us Sicker and Poorer* (New York: Bloomsbury, 2007): 293.

7. Susan B. Foote, *Managing the Medicare Arms Race: Public Policy and Medical Device Innovation* (Berkeley: University of California Press, 1992); Marcia Angell, *The Truth about Drug Companies: How They Deceive Us and What to Do about It* (New York: Random House, 2004); Jerry Avorn, "Rethinking Research Funding,"

Boston Globe, May 7, 2007; Donald L. Bartlett and James B. Steele, *Critical Condition: How Health Care in America Became Big Business—and Bad Medicine* (New York: Doubleday Press, 2004).

8. Anupam B. Jena and Tomas Phillipson, "Cost-Effectiveness as a Price Control," *Health Affairs* 26, no. 3 (2007): 696–703.

9. Richard A. Deyo and Donald L. Patrick, "Hope or Hype: The Obsession with Medical Advances and the High Cost of False Promises," (New York: American Management Association, 2004): 79.

10. Angell, *The Truth About Drug Companies;* Deyo and Patrick, "Hope or Hype"; Avorn, "Rethinking Research Funding"; Bartlett and Steele, *Critical Condition;* Daniel Callahan and Angela Wasunna, *Medicine and the Market: Equity v. Choice* (Baltimore: Johns Hopkins University Press, 2006).

11. Bartlett and Steele, *Critical Condition* 120.

12. Peter Conrad, *The Medicalization of Society* (Baltimore: Johns Hopkins University Press, 2007): 4.

13. Ibid.

14. Ibid., 142.

15. Leonard M. Fleck, "The Costs of Caring: Who Pays? Who Profits? Who Panders?" *Hastings Center Report* 36, no. 3 (2006): 13–17.

16. Avorn, "Rethinking Research Funding."

17. Stephen Heuser, "Tough Criticisms Rise as Biotech Matures," *Boston Globe,* May 8, 2007.

18. Joseph P. Newhouse, "How Much Should Medicare Pay for Drugs?" *Health Affairs* 23, no. 1 (2004): 89–102.

19. Arnold S. Relman, *A Second Opinion: Rescuing America's Health Care* (New York: Public Affairs, 2007): 5.

20. Rosemary A. Stevens, "History and Health Policy in the United States: The Making of a Health Care Industry, 1948–2008" *Social History of Medicine* 21, no. 3: 483.

21. John K. Iglehart, "The Emergence of Physician-Owned Specialty Hospitals," *New England Journal of Medicine* 352, no. 1 (2005): 78–84.

22. Robert A. Berenson, Paul B. Ginsburg, and Jessica H. May, "Hospital–Physician Relations: Cooperation, Competition, or Separation?" *Health Affairs* (Web Exclusive, 2006): W34.

23. Ibid., W41.

24. Jeff Goldsmith, "Hospitals and Physicians: Not a Pretty Picture," *Health Affairs* (Web Exclusive, 2006): W73.

25. Jean M. Mitchell, "The Prevalence of Physician Self-Referral Arrangements after Stark II: Evidence from Advanced Diagnostic Imaging," *Health Affairs* (Web Exclusive 2007): W415–W435.

26. Stephanie Maxwell, Stephen Zuckerman, and Robert A. Berenson, "Use of Physicians' Services under Medicare's Resource-Based Payment," *New England Journal of Medicine* 356, no. 18 (2007): 1853–1861.

27. Ibid., 1853.

28. Newhouse, "How Much Should Medicare Pay for Drugs?"

29. Dana Gelb Safran, "Defining the Future of Primary Care: What Can We Learn from Patients," *Annals of Internal Medicine* 130, no. 3 (2003): 248.

30. Ibid.

31. Ibid., 249.

32. Ibid., 251.

33. Ibid., 253.

34. Thomas Bodenheimer, Robert A. Berenson, and Paul Rudolph, "The Primary Care–Specialty Income Gap—Why It Matters," *Annals of Internal Medicine* 146, no. 4 (2007): 301–306.

35. Thomas Bodenheimer, "Primary Care—Will It Survive?" *New England Journal of Medicine* 355, no. 9 (2006): 862.

36. Beverly Woo, "Primary Care: The Best Job in Medicine," *New England Journal of Medicine* 355, no. 9 (2006): 866.

37. Ibid.

38. Mark A. Rodwin, Hak J. Chang, and Jeffrey Clausen, "Malpractice Premiums and Physicians' Income: Perceptions of a Crisis Conflict with Empirical Evidence," *Health Affairs* 25, no. 1 (2006): 750–758.

39. Jack M. Colwill, James M. Cultice, and Robin L. Kruse, "Will Generalist Physician Supply Meet Demands of an Increasing and Aging Society?" *Health Affairs*, Web Exclusive (April 2008): 232–241.

40. Relman, *A Second Opinion*, 166.

41. Ibid., 170.

CHAPTER 6: "MEDICAL NECESSITY": AN ALL-BUT-USELESS CONCEPT

1. Daniel Callahan, *False Hopes: Overcoming the Obstacles to a Sustainable, Affordable Medicine* (New York: Simon & Schuster, 1998).

2. John A. Vincent, "Science and Imagery in the 'War on Old Age,' " *Aging and Society* 29 (2007): 941–961.

3. René Dubos, *The Mirage of Health: Utopias, Progress, and Biological Change* (New York: Harper Colophon, 1979): 2.

4. Michael Walzer, *Spheres of Justice: A Defense of Pluralism and Equality* (New York: Basic Books, 1983): 88.

5. Daniel Callahan, *Living with Mortality: In Search of a Peaceful Death* (New York: Simon and Schuster, 1993).

6. Daniel Callahan, *What Price Better Health: Hazards of the Research Imperative* (Berkeley: University of California Press, 2003).

7. Jessica H. Miller and Barbara Koenig, "On the Boundary of Life and Death," in *Biomedicine Examined*, ed. Margaret Lock and Deborah Gordon (Dordrecht: Kluwer Academic Publishers, 1988): 369.

8. Christine Overall, *Aging, Death and Human Longevity* (Berkeley: University of California Press, 2003).

9. William Haseltine, quoted in Lawrence M. Fisher, "The Race to Cash in on the Genetic Code," *New York Times*, August 29, 1999.

10. Nicholas Agar, "Whereto Transhumanism?" *Hastings Center Report* 37, no. 3 (2007): 12–17.

11. Geoffrey Scarre, *Death* (Montreal: McGill-Queen's University Press, 2007).

12. Vincent, "Science and Imagery," 941.

13. Seneca, quoted in Scarre, *Death*, 35.

14. Judith Feder and Donald W. Moran, "Cost Containment and the Politics of Health Care Reform," in *Restoring Fiscal Sanity 2007: The Health Spending Challenge,* ed. Alice M. Rivlin and Joseph R. Antos (Washington, D.C.: The Brookings Institution, 2007): 186.

15. Joanne Lynn, *Sick to Death: And Not Going to Take It Anymore* (Berkeley: University of California Press, 2004).

16. Cited in Jacqueline Fox, "Medicare Should, but Cannot, Consider Costs: Legal Impediments to a Sound Policy," *Buffalo Law Review* 53, no. 2 (2005): 590-591.

17. Mark A. Hall, "State Regulation of Medical Necessity: The Case of Weight-Reduction Surgery," *Duke Law Journal* 53 (2003): 671.

18. Ibid., 672.

19. David M. Eddy, "Evidence-Based Medicine: A Unified Approach," *Health Affairs* 24, no. 1 (2005): 9–17.

20. Ibid., 9.

21. James C. Robinson, "The End of Managed Care," *JAMA* 285, no. 20 (2000): 2622.

22. Jean R. Tunis, "Why Medicine Has Not Established Criteria for Coverage Decisions," *New England Journal of Medicine* 350, no. 21 (2004): 2197.

23. Peter J. Neumann, Allison B. Rosen, and Milton C. Weinstein, "Medicare and Cost Effectiveness Analysis," *New England Journal of Medicine* 353, no. 14 (2005): 1519.

24. Jacqueline Fox, "Medicare Should, but Cannot, Consider Cost: Legal Impediments to a Sound Policy," *Buffalo Law Review* 53, no. 2 (2005): 632.

25. Muriel G. Gillick, "Medicare Coverage for Technological Innovations: Time for New Criteria?" *New England Journal of Medicine* 350 (2004): 2199–2203.

26. Ibid., 2201.

27. Peter S. Neumann, Maki S. Kamae, Jennifer A. Palmer, "Medicare's National Coverage Decisions for Technologies, 1999–2007," *Health Affairs* 24, no. 1 (2008): 1620.

28. Tunis, "Why Medicare Has Not Established Criteria," 2197.

29. Ibid., 2198.

30. Fox, "Medicare Should, but Cannot, Consider Cost," 611.

31. David Eddy, quoted in Peter A. Glassman et al., "The Role of Medical Necessity and Cost-Effectiveness in Making Medical Decisions," *Annals of Internal Medicine* 126, no. 2 (1997): 152.

32. Gillick, "Medicare Coverage for Technological Innovations," 2201.

33. Fox, "Medicare Should, but Cannot, Consider Cost."

34. Ibid.

35. Ibid.

36. Ibid., 612.

37. Neumann, Rosen, and Milton, "Medicare and Cost Effectiveness Analysis," 1518.

38. Ibid.

CHAPTER 7: REDEFINING "MEDICAL NECESSITY":
FROM INDIVIDUAL GOOD TO SOCIAL GOOD

1. Thomas E. Getzen, "Health Care Is an Individual Necessity and a National Luxury: Applying Multilevel Decision Models to the Analysis of Health Care Expenditures," *Journal of Health Economics* 19 (2000): 268.

2. Guillem Lopez, personal communication, October 30, 2007.

3. Daniel Callahan, *Setting Limits: Medical Goods in an Aging Society* (New York: Simon & Schuster: 1987).

4. Alexander M. Capron, "Ethical Aspects of Major Increases in Life Span and Life Expectancy," in *Coping with Methuselah: The Impact of Molecular Biology and Society*, ed. Henry J. Aaron and William B. Schwartz (Washington, D.C.: Brookings Institution Press, 2004).

5. Christine Overall, *Aging, Death and Human Longevity* (Berkeley: University of California Press, 2003).

6. John A. Vincent, "Science and Imagery in the 'War on Old Age,'" *Ageing and Society* 27 (2007): 941.

7. Joel Mokyr, *The Lever of Riches: Technological Creativity and Economic Progress* (New York: Oxford University Press, 1990): 210.

8. Barnaby J. Feder, "A Lifesaver, but the Risks Give Pause," *New York Times*, September 13, 2008.

9. Gerald F. Ailey, "Long-Term Trends in the Concentration of Medicare Spending," *Health Affairs* 26, no. 3 (2007): 808–819.

10. Dana P. Goldman et al., "Consequences of Health Trends and Medical Innovation for the Future Elderly," *Health Affairs* 24, suppl. 2 (2005): R5–17.

11. Donald R. Hoover et al., "Medical Expenditures during the Last Year of Life: Findings from the 1992–1996 Medicare Current Beneficiary Survey," *HSR: Health Services Research* 37, no. 6 (2002): 1625–1642; Michael Raitano, "The Impact of Death-Related Costs on Healthcare Expenditure: A Survey," ENEPRI Report no. 17 (2006).

12. Hoover et al., "Medical Expenditures"; James Lubitz, "Health, Technology, and Medical Care Spending," *Health Affairs* 24 (web exclusive, 2005): W81–W85.

13. Meena Seshamahi and Alastair M. Gray, "A Longitudinal Study of the Effects of Age and Time to Death on Hospital Costs," *Journal of Health Economics* 23 (2004): 222–223.

14. Christopher Hogan et al., "Medicare Beneficiaries' Cost of Care in the Last Year of Life," *Health Affairs* 20, no. 4 (2001): 192.

15. Marc L. Berk and Alan C. Monheit, "The Concentration of Health Care Expenditures, Revisited," *Health Affairs* 20, no. 2 (2001): 9–18; Gerald F. Riley, "Long-Term Trends in the Concentration of Medicare Spending," *Health Affairs* 26, no. 3 (2007): 808–819.

16. Berk and Monheit, "The Concentration of Health Care Expenditures, Revisited," 110, 112.

17. Ibid., 112.

18. James Lubitz et al., "Health, Life Expectancy, and Health Care Spending among the Elderly," *New England Journal of Medicine* 249, no. 11 (2003): 1048; Hoover et al., "Medical Expenditures," 1639.

19. Dartmouth Atlas Project, "The Care of Patients with Severe Chronic Illness: A Report on the Medicare Program by the Dartmouth Atlas Project," http://www.dartmouthatlas.org/atlases/2006_Atlas_Exec_Summary.pdf.

20. Ibid., 1.

21. Elliott S. Fisher et al., "The Implications of Regional Variations in Medicare Spending, Part 2: Health Outcomes and Satisfaction with Care," *Annals of Internal Medicine* 138, no. 4 (2003): 288–298.

22. Dartmouth Atlas Project, "The Care of Patients," 2.

23. Daniel Callahan and Angela A. Wasunna, *Medicine and the Market: Equity v. Choice* (Baltimore: Johns Hopkins University Press, 2006).

24. Christopher J. L. Murray et al., "Eight Americas: Investigating Mortality Disparities across Races, Counties, and Race-Counties in the United States," *PLoS Medicine* 3, no. 9 (2006): 1513–1524; David Mechanic, "Population Health: Challenges for Science and Society," *The Milbank Quarterly* 85, no. 3 (2007): 533–559.

25. David A. Kindig takes a somewhat different route to a public health model in "A Pay-for-Population Health Performance," *JAMA* 296, no. 21 (2006).

26. Daniel Callahan, *What Kind of Life: The Limits of Medical Progress* (New York: Simon & Schuster, 1990): 176–177.

27. Michael D. Rawlins and Anthony J. Culyer, "National Institute for Clinical Excellence and Its Value Judgments" *British Medical Journal* 329, no. 7459 (2004): 224.

CHAPTER 8: GETTING OUT FROM UNDER: THE POLITICS OF PAIN

1. Thomas R. Frieden and Farzad Mostashari, "Health Care as if Health Mattered," *JAMA* 299, no. 8 (2008): 950.

2. Shannon Brownlee, *Overtreated: Why Too Much Medicine Is Making Us Sicker and Poorer* (New York: Bloomsbury, 2007).

3. Robin Hanson, "Cut Medicine in Half," Cato Unbound Blog, the Cato Institute, September 10, 2007. http://www.cato-unbound.org/2007/09/10/robin-hanson/cut-medicine-in-half/

4. Ellen Nolte and C. Martin McKee, "Measuring the Health of Nations: Updating an Earlier Analysis," *Health Affairs* (January/February 2008): 98.

5. Karen Schoen et al., "Bending the Curve: Options for Achieving Savings and Improved Value in U.S. Health Spending," *The Commonwealth Fund* 80 (November 18, 2007), *http://www.Commonwealthfund.org/publications/publications_show .htm?doc_id==620087.*

6. Gregg Easterbrook, *The Progress Paradox: How Life Gets Better while People Feel Worse* (New York: Random House, 2003).

7. Arthur J. Barsky, *Worried Sick: Our Troubled Quest for Wellness* (Boston: Little Brown, 1988).

8. Jonathan Cohn, "Creative Destruction: The Best Case against Universal Health Care, *The New Republic* (November 19, 2007), 28.

9. Daniel Callahan, "Advocacy and Priorities for Research," in *What Price Better Health: Hazards of the Research Imperative* (Berkeley: University of California Press, 2006), Chapter 6.

10. Steven H. Woolf, "Potential Health and Economic Consequences of Misplaced Priorities," *JAMA* 29, no. 5 (2007): 523.

11. Richard Dolinar, "Evidence-Based Medicine vs. Patients," *TCS Daily* (December 17, 2007).

12. Samuel H. Preston, "Children and the Elderly: Divergent Paths for America's Dependents," *Demography* 21 (1984): 491.

13. Daniel Callahan, *Setting Limits: Medical Goals in an Aging Society* (New York: Simon & Schuster, 1987).

CODA

1. Gardiner Harris, "British Balance Benefit vs. Cost of Latest Drugs," *The New York Times*, December 3, 2008: A1.

2. K. Robin Yabroff, et al., "Projections of Costs Associated with Colorectal Cancer Care in the United States," *Health Economics* 17 (2008): 955.

3. Ibid, 955.

4. K. Robin Yaroff, et al. "Cost of Care for Elderly Cancer Patients in the United States, *Journal of the National Cancer Institute* 100, no. 9 (2008): 640.

INDEX

Aaron, Henry, 43, 55, 85
AARP Public Policy Institute report (2008), 21
ACP Journal Club, 59
ADHD (attention-deficit/hyperactivity disorder), 128
Advanced Medical Technology Association (AdvaMed), 124
advocacy constituency, 220–21
Agency for Health Care Policy and Research, 123
Agency for Health Care Quality and Research, 124
aging, biomedicalized conception of, 49
American College of Cardiology, 53
American College of Radiology, 53
American culture: choice and individualism values of, 143–44; commitment to medical industry in, 121–22; health care reform and role of, 81–82; health obsession of, 154–55; love of commerce as part of, 120; medical industry clash of values within, 140; medical technology love by, 90–91, 120; value on making money in, 140–41. *See also* United States; values
American Federation of Government Employees (AFGE), 103
American Medical Association (AMA): market-based approach to health insurance by, 73; Medicare passage opposition by, 12; National Center for Health Care Technology opposition by, 122. *See also* medical industry
antiplatet therapy, 43
Antos, Joseph R., 65, 66
Armey, Dick, 27
Arrow, Kenneth, 93–94
Avastin, 131
Avorn, Jerry, 131

baby boom generation: European vs. U.S. approach to, 26; later adulthood (36–70

years) health care, 188–90; projecting Medicare enrollment by, 14; proposed Medicare buy-in for, 71. *See also* elderly population
Baltimore hospital competition study (1971–1990), 99–100
Barsky, Arthur, 208
Bartlett, Donald L., 128
basic package. *See* health care basic package
Baucus, Max, 116
Bayh, Birch, 127
behavioral incentives programs, 57–58
Bemazai, Anil, 98
beneficiary costs: out-of-pocket, 2, 12–13; proposed increase of, 19
Berenson, Robert A., 135
Berk, Mark L., 184
Biogen Idec, 131
"biomedicalized conception of aging," 49
biotechnology industry, 130–31
Biotechnology Industry Organization (BIO), 124
Blair, Tony, 108
Bodenheimer, Thomas, 99, 137
Bokhari, Farasat, 102
Bourdelais, Patrice, 42
British National Institute for Clinical Excellence (NICE), 199–200, 211, 231
Brownlee, Sarah, 205–6
Brownlee, Shannon, 123
Buckley, Edward, 101
Bush administration (1989–1993), 26–28
Bush administration (2000–2008), 14, 16, 40–41
Bush, George W., 16
The Business of Health (Ohsfeldt and Schneider), 111
Butler, Stuart, 95–96

Canada: comparative study of supply-side constraints on care in, 77–78; competitive

Thatcher, Margaret, 108
third-party payments, 141
Thomas, Lewis, 22
Town, Robert J., 98
transhumanism movement, 152, 180
Truman administration, 12
Tunis, Sean, 164, 165, 166

UK (United Kingdom): comparison between
The Netherlands and, 109; control of infla-
tion rates in, 33; National Health Service
of, 200, 211–12; National Institute for
Clinical Excellence (NICE) of the, 199–
200, 211, 231; universal coverage/competi-
tion balance in, 108–9
"Uncertainty and the Welfare Economics of
Medical Care" (Arrow), 93–94
United Health Foundation, 84
The United State National Insurance Act
(Medicare for All) [HR 676] bill, 78–79, 80
United States: aging societies approach by
Europe vs., 26; comparative per capita for
health care costs in the, 78; comparative
study of supply-side constraints in the,
77–78; control of pharmaceuticals in the,
76–77; eliminating health care inequities
in the, 186; failure of health care competition in the, 109–12; health care costs as
outpacing GDP of the, 1, 35, 38–39; highest life expectancy rates of over 80 years
by the, 28; percentage increase in health
care costs (1970–2004) in the, 111t; periodic health care crises in the, 1; public
opinion survey on medical technology interest in, 48–49; rate of annual health care
cost inflation in, 39. See also American
culture
universal health care system: Canadian policy outlawing private care outside of, 193;
conciliatory track toward, 228; cost control issues for, 5, 209–10; failed Truman administration proposals for, 12; government-managed competition and, 105–9,
117–19; health care vouchers proposal for,
30, 73–74; public opinion on degree of support for, 81; Senator Wyden's proposal
for, 72
University of California at Los Angeles
(UCLA) Hospital, 185
University of California San Francisco Medical Center, 185
unmet needs, 185–86

Urban Institute, 218
U.S. Panel on Cost-Effectiveness in Health
and Medicine, 87

"value for money" concept, 82–85, 169. See
also cost-effectiveness standard
values: choice and individualism, 143–44;
health care reform in context of, 7; health
care and underlying social and economic,
148; medical industry and clash of, 140; pa-
tient-self-definition decisions based in,
143–44; shaping consensus on personal
health policy, 155–57; shaping our personal health care, 148–49. See also American culture; values
VA (Veteran's Administration), 124, 132,
209
Vermont VA Outcomes Group, 51
Viagra, 91
Vincent, John A., 153
Vistnes, G., 98
Vladeck, Bruce, 35–40
Volpe, Kevin G., 101

Wall Street Journal, 27
Wall Street Journal/Harris poll (2006), 20
Wal-Mart treatment facilities, 186, 212, 227
Walzer, Michael, 147
war against cancer (1970), 150
Washington, George, 152
Weisbrod, Burton, 94
Welch, Gilbert, 51–52
wellness programs, 57–58
Wennberg, John, 23–24, 184, 205, 211
"What's Making Us Sick is an Epidemic of
Diagnoses" (Welch), 51–52
White, Joseph, 25–26, 32, 110
White, Richard, 42
"whole person" orientation, 136–37
Woo, Beverly, 137–38
Wood, Alastair J., 43
Woolf, Steven H., 212
World Health Organization study (2004), 33
World Health Organization study (2008), 83
Worried Sick: Our Troubled Quest for Well-
ness (Barsky), 208
Wyden, Ron, 72

young adulthood (18–35 years) health
care, 188

Zwanziger, Jack, 98, 100

Lightning Source UK Ltd.
Milton Keynes UK
UKOW01f1100260218

318485UK00003B/533/P

9 780691 177991